# The New Medicine Man

*A Different Kind of
Health Care for the Elderly*

HUGH A. SCOTT

FITHIAN PRESS
SANTA BARBARA · 1992

Cover by Ren Wicks, Group West, Los Angeles
Design and typography by Jim Cook

LIBRARY OF CONGRESS CATALOGING-IN-PUBLICATION DATA
Scott, Hugh A., 1913–
    The new medicine man: a different kind of health care for
the elderly / Hugh A. Scott.
      p.  cm.
    Includes biographical references.
    ISBN 1-56474-004-8
    1. Aged—Medical care. 2. Holistic medicine. I. Title.
RA564.8.S4  1992                       91-24245
362.1'9897—dc 20                     CIP

The author gratefully acknowledges permission to reprint extracts from the following works:

*Feeling Better* by Larry Feldman. Reprinted with the permission of the author.

*Science and Creation* by John Polkinghorne, ©1988 by John Polkinghorne. Reprinted by arrangement with Shambhala Publications, Inc., 300 Massachusetts Ave., Boston, MA 02115.

*The Tao of Physics* by Fritjof Capra, ©1983 by Fritjof Capra. Reprinted by arrangement with Shambhala Publications, Inc., 300 Massachusetts Ave., Boston, MA 02115.

*The Brain in Human Aging* by Gene D. Cohen, ©1988. Reprinted by permission of Springer Publishing Co., Inc., New York, NY 10012

*Mind as Healer, Mind as Slayer* by Dr. Kenneth Pelletier. Reprinted by permission of Delacorte Press, New York, NY 10103.

"Ministers Under Stress" by Hank Whittemore. Reprinted with permission from Parade Publications, ©1991.

"Last Word" by Ann Ray Martin. Reprinted by permission of Longevity, ©1991, Longevity International, Ltd.

*Teach Only Love* by Gerald G. Jampolsky, M.D., Claire Huff. ©1983 by Gerald G. Jampolsky, M.D. Used by permission of Bantam Books, a division of Bantam Doubleday Dell Publishing Group, Inc.

*Health for the Whole Person,* edited by Arthur Hastings, James Fadiman, and James Gordon. Reprinted by permission of the authors.

*Getting Well Again* by Dr. Carl O. Simonton, Jeremy P. Tarcher, Inc.

*The Road Less Traveled* by M. Scott Peck, M.D., ©1978 by M. Scott Peck, M.D. Reprinted by permission of Simon & Schuster, Inc.

*The Turning Point* by Dr. Fritjof Capra, ©1981 by Dr. Fritjof Capra. Reprinted by permission of Simon & Schuster, Inc.

*Love Medicine and Miracles* by Dr. Bernie Siegel, ©by B.H. Siegel, S. Korman, and A. Schiff, Trustees of the Bernard S. Siegel, M.D., Children's Trust. Reprinted by permission of Harper Collins Publishers.

"The Corporate Compromise" by Dr. David Himmelstein and Dr. Steffie Woolhandler in *The Annals of Internal Medicine,* v. 109 (18.9.88): 494. ©American College of Physicians.

The "Dear Abby" column by Abigail Van Buren, ©1990. Reprinted with permission of Universal Press Syndicate.

*To all seekers after truth . . . of whatever age . . .
of whatever time and place . . . of whatever degree
or station in life . . . this book is humbly dedicated.*

# Contents

## Part IV: The Century of the Spirit

# Preface

I'm mad as I write this preface. Mad as in angry. I hadn't planned to write it, but I think I must, because it says a lot about my motivation for writing. Maybe everything that has to be said.

This morning I was out in my front yard, getting in some much-needed weeding. My wife called me in to answer the phone. I felt a twinge of resentment, because I don't like to be interrupted when I'm working outside, any more than I like being interrupted when I'm working at my desk.

Darlene was on the line. Poor gal. She'll be seventy-six in two or three months, and her life is hell right now. It's because of anxiety and panic attacks, mainly, although she has some minor health problems as well.

Darlene first called several months ago, shortly after I'd appeared on television to talk about my getting off drugs. She had similar problems, and thought maybe I could help her. I gave her what encouragement and advice I could, including taking a hard look at her medication, and getting in touch with Karen Mahan to see about biofeedback and mentation counseling. Karen had done the same for me nine years earlier, and had kept me straightened out ever since.

After a lot of calling back and forth, talking to Karen and

changing doctors, getting into treatment with a former student of Karen's and so forth, it had come down to this: Darlene's new doctor was all for the biofeedback, and had even hired the former student to do the biofeedback and mental counseling in his office; the program was working smoothly, but a big hitch developed—the treatment wasn't covered by Medicare.

So what was I supposed to do? I don't have a diploma or any other piece of paper that gives me permission to do anything. I just told Darlene that if she wanted to get herself straightened out, she'd better get over to Karen's and start a program, even if she wound up paying for it herself. If she could get her doctor's permission, so much the better; she might eventually get reimbursed. My own treatment in 1981 was finally covered in full by Medicare, but only because one key symptom was included in my doctor's admitting diagnosis. Medicare won't tell you what these key words are, but if they're not in the diagnosis, forget reimbursement.

This telephone conversation lasted twenty minutes, after which I went back outside and finished weeding, even though I was no longer in the right frame of mind about it.

Why didn't I welcome this opportunity to be of support to a fellow human being? Why do I resent these interruptions, which are happening with increasing frequency these days? It's not because I'm mad at the Darlenes who need help, but because I'm mad at the society, the culture, the public mind-set, the legislation, the bureaucracy, everything that makes it necessary for the Darlenes of the world to go outside any normal, sensible channels to get relief from anxiety and tension, and a lot of other things. If I told you that fear of the unknown, mainly fear of what happens at the time of death and beyond, is behind these widespread and debilitating ailments, you might not believe me, but it's true. That fear and many others as well.

If that were all, and Darlene were the only person on my calling list, I wouldn't be writing this book, because I could handle it with personal contact. But in nearly two years of research—of reading more than forty books, doing at least fifty interviews with highly qualified and competent people, and talking to scores of others who have a pretty good handle on things—I find that the problems are pervasive, touch just about everyone, and have critical relevance for citizens of all age groups, especially the baby boomers who are getting into the really tense period of their lives.

So I think I have a right to ask, why me? Am I special? Why isn't somebody else doing this ? A few are, but they're scattered and pretty much unconnected. Here's some more evidence of the pervasiveness of the problem:

❧ Why does Doris K, a marvelous lady of seventy-five, sit at home and tremble with an uncontrollable nervous tic caused by heavy stress on the job some thirty years ago? She has been misdiagnosed, mismedicated, neglected by her children, and forgotten by society, even though she lives in a beautiful townhouse literally cheek-by-jowl with her intelligent and caring neighbors. They can't read her plight, and find it uncomfortable to be around her. Her doctor is doing his best for her, but it isn't working, and what will work is not covered by Medicare.

❧ Why, at the present moment, are three of my very closest male friends and former associates falling apart from depression, absence of any apparent reason for living, or going through a horrendous divorce and custody procedure? These people are top-drawer by any measure—a former highly respected advertising executive, an internationally known academic, and a youthful publisher on the brink of middle age. All are "in counseling" with psychiatrists and two are on medication, so why do they come to me for help?

❧ Why does my friend, Jean Dunlop, a nurse who runs an alcohol and chemical dependency program for a large hospital, complain that seniors with medication problems won't (or at least don't) come into her program because neither they nor their doctors understand that they are dependent on prescription medications that are bound to let them down if they keep taking them long enough?

❧ Why have I heard personal horror stories about pills from people you'd think would have all the answers, but have missed being able to prevent their own fathers and mothers from going down the mismedication tube? These are not just anybody. The four I'm talking about include a perceptive and widely read author who runs a respected healing center; a nuclear physicist who graduated from the University of California and who is in touch with research efforts nation-wide; the director of a very large medical research laboratory; and a professor of pharmacology at a major medical univer-sity. What can I tell these people?

❡ Why does the most revealing condemnation of our medical and pharmaceutical care come from people closest to the care system itself? If you think I exaggerate, read the work of Drs. William Simonson and Helene Levens Lipton, both of whom wrote books on medication and the elderly, or listen to Dr. John Thompson, director of the Kaiser Permanente Regional Medical Laboratory in Portland, Oregon, and a student of medical culture.

❡ Why do many of the large health maintenance organizations (HMOs) patronize their own members with jolly talk and stories about healthy, active seniors, when so many of their members are sliding down the chute of emotional and spiri-tual dissolution?

❡ Wouldn't you be alarmed if you stood behind an elderly woman at your prescription counter, and heard the clerk tell her that the first supply of pills on her new prescription would cost her $130 for the first month? (I've just read about a breakthrough discovery of a new medication for a rare disease, the only drawback being that the patient will have to pay $300 per month for these pills. A real Catch-22!)

❡ What would you think if a close friend of yours fell off a ladder while painting his house, and died six months later after running up medical and hospital bills of more than $600,000? Should the public pay for this? Or for the high-tech organ transplants and other procedures that can keep people alive, or even "heal" them, when there may be better ways of dealing with their problems?

❡ Am I resentful of the calls for help because I don't want to take the time to answer them, or because it's so hard to find mean-ingful support from all the health care and social agencies that are supposed to be doing this? Am I obligated to lead these care teams—one for each friend or stranger who asks—simply because there's no one else to turn them over to?

Enough. I'm writing this because I want to engage your attention for my analysis of this whole elder health enterprise, and to suggest some solutions that may surprise some people and anger some people, but may give some ideas and hope to a few.

Those of you who have read this far doubtless have a fair idea of who the audiences for this book are. Because these audiences have different interests and viewpoints, they will be more concerned with some parts and chapters than others. However, if you identify with any of the groups I am about to discuss, you should find considerable substance of importance to you if you read far enough. And if you read through to the end, you may gain an idea of the relatedness of many of these problems that you have not previously held.

There are five principal audiences of immediate concern. They are:
1. Primary caregivers to the elderly—spouses, brothers and sisters, and adult children who need a broad and realistic view of the sometimes monumental problems that confront them.
2. Support personnel in the health care field, such as employees in hospital senior service departments, public health and social service workers, physicians' nurses and others doing liaison work with older patients, referral sources such as psychologists, counselors and therapists, employees in state and local senior agencies, and so on.
3. Public officials charged with planning and implementing programs involving senior health care, including office-holders.
4. Other non-profit agencies, religious organizations, etc., which include services to the aging in their portfolios.
5. The elderly themselves, many of whom are competent to manage their own care.

The concept of this book is simple. I had been researching the problem of medication and health care for older people when, about a year and a half ago, it suddenly became very clear to me that there is a huge gap in the services now available for such care.

On the one hand is the traditional medical establishment, which diagnoses and treats physical ailments. On the other hand are the psychologists, counselors, and ministers who deal, in a somewhat fragmented way, with mental, emotional, and spiritual problems.

But for the elders who are alone, depressed, fearful, or anxious, there is often no one to visit them, counsel them, and then find the resources they need to remain functional, or better, to be healed. The farther I pursued the subject, the clearer it became that there is a crying need for a new kind of senior peer counselor to fill this gap, an "elder statesman" type who can link the patient with all the varying support functions, and when necessary, *create* the kind of service that will stabilize a situation or turn it around.

I have designated the prototype of this senior peer counselor the New Medicine Man. You will find an expanded discussion of these perceptions and recommendations in Part II of this book.

I can't tell you where you are most likely to find the "nuggets" of information that will be most helpful to your own thinking. A nugget to one person might be a lump of clay to another. But for each, there should be ideas and examples that are enlightening and useful. You won't get the whole picture unless you read the whole book—all four parts.

I hope the book you are holding becomes well used, with underlinings, highlighting, and scribbled notes. Over time, you'll be able to add many points of your own to the various lists and functional setups I describe. Perhaps if you read the book carefully and take the right notions to heart, you'll even enjoy some of the mental and spiritual growth that I experienced in researching and writing it.

Good reading!

# Acknowledgments

It's commonplace that authors of books of research and opinion acknowledge the contributions of other writers and researchers in getting their material together, but in the case of myself and the book you have in hand, this is not just a moral obligation, but an imminent necessity. Until about two years ago, I wasn't much more than a babe in the woods when it came to the issues I discuss, and concerning which I have developed (and express) some pretty strong opinions. I must therefore give a major share of credit to a number of people who have not only provided much of my factual material, but who have also shared their views on the major issues involved, who have shown me the safe stepping stones across the river of literature and current information available, and who have warned against some of the most treacherous shoals and eddies.

Of some fifty people I have interviewed, three have been especially helpful, not only because of their professional stature and expertise, but also because they have opened doors to other important sources. They are Dr. Merwyn (Mitch) Greenlick, director of the Kaiser Permanente Center for Health Research in Portland; Dr. John Thompson, director of the Kaiser Permanente Regional Laboratory, also in Portland; and Dr. Charles Strother, a psychologist and former corporate president of Group Health Cooperative of Puget Sound, in Seattle. With the interest and active support of such as these, I could pursue my inquiries with dispatch and peace of mind, because I could avoid blind alleys and gain critical information with a minimum of wasted time and effort.

All of those whom I interviewed, or from whom I received information in response to inquiries, are listed in Appendix B in the back of this book. I should make note here of a few who provided information and suggestions beyond the answers requested. They are:

—Joe Adams, former assistant dean at the Oregon Health Sciences University, who has many friends in the medical fraternity, as well as a wealth of background in the way things have happened and are happening in health care;

—Dr. Joyce Colling, a registered nurse and professional gerontologist, who served on the American Nurses Association committee monitoring federal legislation in the nursing home field;

—Jean Dunlop, RN, experienced in alcohol and drug rehabilitation for the elderly, who assisted in planning and putting on a symposium on medication and the elderly;

—Dr. Michael Fleming, a psychologist with experience in getting elders off drugs, who also has a highly developed social consciousness;

—Sally Goodwin, director of the Oregon Association of Homes for the Aging, who gave me valuable insights in current trends in nursing home management;

—Rev. Greg Ikehara-Martin, who provided definitive background on the Stephen Ministries movement, as well as suggestions for further research;

—Dr. Gerry Jampolsky, author of *Teach Only Love,* who took the time to write me his views on the relation of love to the conquest of fear in healing;

—Dr. Phyllis McGraw, a clinical psychologist, who conferred with me several times on the psychological problems of elders relative to spiritual issues;

—Lucy Nonnenkamp, who supervises the Social/HMO pro-

*Acknowledgments*

gram for Kaiser Permanente, for backgrounding me on the current status of that important Medicare initiative;
—Dee Pennock, a writer on health issues, for sharing many of her manuscripts and contacts with me;
—Dr. Edward Rosenbaum, a Portland rheumatologist and author, for counseling me both on medical and publishing matters;
—Marv Rosenberg of Group Health Cooperative of Puget Sound, for giving me critical information and opinions concerning his group's pioneering work with senior peer counselors;
—Dr. William Simonson, professor of pharmacology at Oregon State University, for his confidence in asking me to participate in a panel on medication and the elderly at the 1991 conference of the National Council on Aging in Miami;
—Dorothy Sullivan, RN, director of a Catholic parish program for counseling and assisting the elderly-aged in her parish, for access to seminars and discussions with her peers;
—Claire Wart, RN, for providing a model of community health care for the elderly, and taking part in my symposium on medication.

Also, a special thanks for backup and ideas in many areas of my investigation to Chuck Keaty and Jay Gusick of Group Health Coop of Puget Sound; to Jim Samuels and Karen Mahan for dozens of classes and consultations in mentation and personal development; and to William Van Bise and Dr. Elizabeth Rauscher for technical and scientific input in a number of areas.

Finally, I take off my hat to Ren Wicks, a well known commercial artist in Los Angeles, who designed and executed the cover of this book. Ren, whom I have known since we were in school together in 1924, is a founding member of the Aviation Artists Association of America, and has created ten commemorative stamps for the Postal Service, among other important commissions.

Every day, I have reason to be thankful for new contacts, new sources of information, and new support. There's not room here for all, but my heartfelt appreciation anyway!

# The New Medicine Man

# Prologue

On the morning of February 12, 1991, I sat in the apartment of Dr. Charles Strother, a psychologist and one of the founders of Group Health Cooperative of Puget Sound, on the fourteenth floor of the Park Shore retirement center in Seattle, overlooking Lake Washington. I had driven up from Portland, Oregon, especially to see him, because I knew he had strong views about the need for new methods of dealing with the health care of the elderly, paralleling many conclusions I had reached myself.

Dr. Strother had sent me some briefing papers on this subject, and had written two long letters in which he developed his opinions. His cooperative, a health maintenance organization or HMO, now enrolls 440,000 persons of all ages in Washington and a few in Oregon, including a self-governing subsidiary in Spokane. It is the largest cooperative HMO in the United States, and has been a pioneer in many fields of group care. Dr. Strother had concluded one of his letters with this paragraph:

> We need a new look at geriatric care—a look that will take into consideration the unique characteristics and needs of geriatric patients, a look that will recognize the important differences between geriatric medicine and general medicine; a plan that will provide the staffing patterns and treatment resources that will be required; and a plan that will be based on the appropriate principles of geriatric care.

I could have said, "You're singing my song, Chuck," because those words echoed exactly what I had been thinking, saying, and writing for the past year. But I didn't say this, because our conversation soon led us into an area of disagreement.

Basically, Dr. Strother's argument was that for his new model to be properly recognized and funded and to serve an appreciable number of people, it would have to be built into an organizational structure like Group Health. It would have to be based on a comprehensive plan providing health maintenance and prevention of illness, as well as care in the doctor's office, in the home, in the community, in hospitals, and in all types of long-term care facilities, even at life's end through hospice services. This would require an extensive process of planning and implementation.

My argument was the mirror image of this. I told him that his idea was fine for a large organization such as Group Health, which has the resources, the staff, the offices, and the buildings and personnel to take care of its half-million patients. But I pointed out that there are millions of other people who do not have access to his kind of service, or who choose to go some other route. They may be lonely, depressed, and confused. A lot of them don't know how to handle their medical insurance, or even to tell whether the care they are getting is as good as it should be. They often feel abandoned, and resign themselves to living in fear and ignorance between visits to their doctor's office. I proposed that we start at the grassroots with small ad hoc teams, with volunteer support that simply begins doing what needs to be done.

Dr. Strother gave me a sharp glance, and finally said, "We're approaching this problem from two entirely different levels—I'm approaching it from the top down, and you're doing it from the bottom up!"

I had to agree with him, but I wasn't quick enough to state the obvious—there is no reason why people in position to take some action on this problem can't begin to work on both approaches simultaneously, because they are not mutually exclusive. I'll develop my thoughts in the following chapter, and will present more of Dr. Strother's thinking toward the end of Part I.

# Part I:
# New Times,
# New Models

❡ *You have to go into the homes where the elderly are, if you are going to find them and give them any kind of help.*

# 1. How I Became a Caregiver

Full dark had descended on the western slope of the Coast Range of Oregon in the late afternoon of November 9, 1965. On top of that, the rain was coming down in gusty sheets, sweeping in from the ocean in relentless torrents characteristic of our winter storms.

My father was driving his dark green Chevrolet station wagon from his home at Neah-Kah-Nie, overlooking the ocean, back to Portland on the Sunset Highway, U.S. 26. With him in the front seat was Ned Fulton, a visiting friend. In the back seat were Mother, on the left side, and Ned's wife, Alla Bess, who had been injured in an automobile accident earlier in the day.

When the Fultons had reached my parents' home after a delay caused by that wreck, Dad had insisted on driving Alla Bess to a hospital in Portland, eighty-four miles away. His car had reached Milepost 26, eastbound, just four miles east of a well-known landmark, Elderberry Inn, when the way was blocked by another vehicle—a low-boy trailer carrying a large piece of construction equipment. Evidence indicates that the trailer and its towing unit were going about twelve miles an hour. Dad was doing about fifty.

Other drivers who were following Dad's car told state police that Dad's brake lights never came on. It is believed that his Chevrolet hit the low-boy and its load without slowing down, shoving the car's engine halfway back into the driver's compartment, and smashing both front fender panels and the bumper assembly.

Dad's chest was crushed against the steering column. He was dead on arrival at St. Vincent Hospital in Portland about an hour later. Ned Fulton's head went into the windshield, and he, likewise, was dead when he reached a hospital in Seaside, Oregon, on the Oregon coast. Mother was taken to St. Vincent in the same ambulance as Dad; she had a fractured skull and right femur, and many other injuries. Alla Bess Fulton's jaw had been broken in the earlier accident, and now her knees had been smashed in addition to multiple lacerations and other injuries. She was taken to Seaside.

My wife, Erma, and I were at home in northeast Portland when we received a call from St. Vincent, in the northwest part of Portland, seven miles away. We reached there sometime after 7 P.M., and were told the situation by Dr. Charles Fagan, an orthopedic surgeon who, by great good fortune, had been at the hospital at the time my parents were brought in. He took charge of my mother's case, and with skillful surgery and continued supervision, helped to restore her to mobility and a measure of life enjoyment.

I viewed my father's body at the hospital, and next day, with Erma, made arrangements for the funeral, and began all the other notifications and terminal processes.

Thus, without advance notice or the least expectation, Erma and I became caregivers for the first time in our lives. We had had no preparation for this: no classes, no reading material, no support group, no consultation, no planning, no chance to ascertain our patient's wishes. Mother had been conscious but irrational during her first eleven days in the hospital. She didn't even know where she was until one afternoon, when I visited her after work, and she pressed me as to where my father was and why she hadn't seen him. I judged she was ready for the news; I told her that he had died in the same accident that had caused her injuries. It was as though I had thrown a light switch. Mother made an immediate connection with reality, and didn't let it go until she died more than five years later.

It is not my intention in this book to write in any detail about my own experiences as a caregiver. I'll say, however, that taking care of Mother and her affairs was just an introduction to the whole world of caring for the elderly, and I have had occasion to take part in, or to observe, more than a dozen caregiving situations involving family or close friends in the ensuing years. These included the final years of Erma's father and stepmother, who were placed in a nursing home together in 1977. Her stepmother survived only three weeks in the nursing home, but her father lived four more years, during which we visited him monthly or more often.

These experiences and the many observations I made, the conclusions I've drawn, and the research I've undertaken have led me to put this book together. My hope is that it will have value for three broad groups of people: first, those who, like Erma and me, have been thrown into the role of caregiver without prior planning or preparation; second, the professionals, paraprofessionals, and volunteers who give them close support; and third, the public and private agencies and organizations that place a priority on giving adequate care to our growing population of elderly.

I have tried to stay close to a sound rationale in reporting my findings, but expect that many of these will be controversial; others will work for some people but not for others. My emphasis is on individual enterprise and effort, and on organization from the bottom up rather than from the top down. Some portions of the field are already served by existing community groups and agencies, but even these do not always cover all the bases, and may be restricted by lack of funds. Readers are free to borrow as heavily as they wish from my suggestions, to tailor them to their own requirements, and to make improvements as they see fit. The only failure, in my view, will be the failure to try *something* or to do more than is now being done for seniors who have lost the means to do these things for themselves.

# 2. New Times, New Models

If you live in an urban community of whatever size anywhere in the United States, the chances are great that, within a block or two of your home, there is at least one elderly person who suffers from a lack of some kind of care. These people are both silent and invisible, as far as the public is concerned. Their needs are myriad, but caregivers and social workers generally will recognize the following conditions as typical:

• **Loneliness and depression.** These go together, like hot dogs and mustard. They are lonely because spouses have died, children live at a distance (or simply fail to visit or call), former friends have also died or moved away, and neighbors have never gotten to know them. They are the ones who have given up community activities because of failing health or because they were not the spouse who took the lead in these matters.

• **Incompetence and confusion.** These also go together. Few people realize the extent to which couples develop a division of labor over a lifetime of marriage. One brings home the bacon, takes care of financial matters, does the yard work and house maintenance, keeps the car running, and makes the economic decisions. The other buys the groceries, does the housework, keeps up with correspondence and communications with relatives and friends, cooks the meals, and deals with repairmen and shopkeepers. These roles vary from couple to couple, but they all have to be performed by someone in a well-functioning marriage. When either spouse dies or is permanently incapacitated, the other has a double burden—all of his or her former functions, plus those of the non-functioning spouse. Too often, the survivor is totally unprepared to take over these unfamiliar duties, and either has to learn the hard way or get someone else to take them over.

• **Hypochondria and/or chronic illness.** The headline in a recent news article said: "Hypochondria, far from being laughable, is abnormal behavior that can hide other serious mental problems." Hypochondria is as disabling as any real illness; but many elders, faced with the stress of loneliness, depression, incompetence, and confusion, slide into chronic illness—real or imagined—to compensate for their lack of ability to deal with life's problems.

But do you think these disabling stresses, which form the real core of the health care needs of our seniors, are being adequately addressed? Hardly; if they were, there would be no need for this book. Rather, the contemporary approach to medicine, championed and administered by medical doctors, has been to diagnose and treat physical ailments germ by germ, body part by body part. The role of the mind is acknowledged, but among doctors, this area of health care has been assigned to psychiatrists, who are MDs specializing in mental illness. Like other MDs, psychiatrists are trained to diagnose and treat the diseases of their patients. Too often, their treatment touches only the symptoms they are able to diagnose, without reaching more deeply buried problems.

The role of government in the health care of seniors has been grossly overemphasized. Medicare has become not only the tail that wags the dog, it is the dog and tail together. In recent years, due to vast pressures from the public, from Congress, from business and labor organizations, and other users of health care services, Medicare administrators have tried to curtail costs through DRGs (Diagnosis Related Groups) defining allowable hospital costs, and have pressed doctors to accept assignment of Medicare benefits as their full compensation for specific patient services. As one result, many doctors have given up treating elderly patients for illnesses that are not adequately covered by Medicare allowances. This is in addition to patients whose symptoms are not found on the charts of diagnostic procedure codes at all. The result has been chaos or stalemate, depending on one's point of view, and has contributed to the mounting chorus of demands for health care reform.

In the course of my reading, interviews, and introspection concerning the wellsprings of healing, I have concluded that when the primary motive of any treatment program is financial profit, healing is greatly inhibited. I made this comment to my friend, Dr. Edward Rosenbaum of Portland, Oregon, and his response was, "If I were in a doctor's examining room, and he left the room to take a call from his stockbroker, I'd walk out the door."

One result of these attitudes is that care for non-physical ailments and all but a handful of non-physical diagnoses that psychiatrists are permitted to make lies wholly outside the model that now governs health care for senior citizens nationally.

Our population of such seniors (those over sixty-five), now numbering nearly forty million, deserves a kind of health care that differs from that of younger people and from what these seniors are now getting.

The true major health needs that grow out of the natural aging process are virtually ignored. Attention is addressed almost exclusively to the symptoms of these ailments, while the pervasive problems of depression, anxiety, a long list of fears and phobias, and failing mental and spiritual faculties go untreated. As a result, no care whatever is provided until patients become physically ill, and then it is often too late to promote healing and restore any degree of quality of life.

The elderly are offered few options between dying ill, miserable, and lonely in their own residences, or dying in care centers that, at best, live up to the title of "nursing homes," but, at worst, are little more than warehouses for the drugged zombies who inhabit them.

The appointment books of most doctors are crowded with patients of all ages, the elderly being accorded only the fifteen minutes each by the standard office schedule. This leaves almost no time for talk and discussion of problems.

Doctors are not adequately educated to treat older people. Typically, medical students take only one course in geriatrics and one in pharmacology. There is relatively little interest among students in geriatrics as a specialty, partly because the doctors do not feel so well-compensated for the time involved, and partly because they dislike the talk-talk they get from lonely, confused elders.

The elderly are often disadvantaged by lower incomes and increased costs of health care, which may not be covered by Medicare or other insurance.

The elderly suffer more than younger persons from health hazards in the home—such as fire danger from stoves and heaters, electrical appliances, cigarettes, and so forth—as well as falls, sprains and fractures, and other causes.

Ills of the elderly in nursing homes are often subject to additive diagnoses; that is, once a diagnosis is placed on a patient's chart, it tends to stay there, even after the symptoms have disappeared.

As people approach old age, they often reach a point at which they suffer from multiple systems failures; that is, they do not regain the function of one organ until another one begins to break down, and this cycle becomes irreversible when enough of a patient's vital functions become seriously weakened.

Like multiple failures of the physical systems, emotional factors such as loneliness, depression, or loss of support from a spouse or other person may pile up until the elderly patients simply lose their will to live.

Cultural differences between generations sometimes make it difficult for younger workers in hospitals, nursing homes, and doctors' offices to relate to the problems of older patients and to communicate effectively with them. Counselors in group therapy programs report that older members are uncomfortable in settings that include younger folk with their casual behavior, four-letter words, and familiar forms of address.

On top of all those factors, add the special problems of diet, incontinence, inability to bathe, reach, dress, carry small items, and so on, and you will understand why most models of care-giving institutions for the elderly are not only outdated but seriously flawed.

It would be a fairly simple matter to design and advocate better ways of taking care of seniors if all other aspects of our health care policies were in good order, but this is not the case. Rather, our national health care system is on a collision course with disaster, and it will avail us little to repattern our senior care system if we fail to deal with the overall problem. The case has been well put by Dr. Ernest Saward, medical director of the northwest region of the Kaiser Permanente health maintenance organization from 1947 to 1970. In March 1989, in the first of the series of annual lectures named for him, he said:

For health care in America, these are the best of times and worst of times. The technology is superb, the expenditure horrendous. . . .

We simply cannot stay as we are. The perception of that fact is quite widespread—and the word *transition* is ubiqui-tous. Transition to what?

Health care expenditures have grown from one-twen-tieth of our nation's gross national product in 1960 to more than one-ninth at the present time. The economic sages indicate further growth in the next ten years to one-seventh of the gross national product (GNP). The chief causes cited to explain this inexorable increase are the aging of the population and the technological imperative. Of course, there are many other causes.

But despite our having the highest costs of any nation, our national health outcome statistics—infant mortality, life expectancy, or any other readily measurable indices—are far from the best. . . .

Our attitude toward the problems of an aging popula-tion, as reflected in the media, often borders on hysteria. But in nations with health outcomes at least equal to or better than ours and with expenditures not only less, but less rapidly increasing, the present fifteen-sixteen percent of the population over sixty-five years does not produce the anxiety that the mere prediction two decades hence does here in the United States. . . .

We are still in an open-ended resource commitment to health care, hence its ever-larger share of our national economy. At some point, however, competing priorities must prevail. . . . Hence the urgent need to change from [this] open-ended resources commitment to health. . . . Change we must. The question is how and when. . . .

America has, in addition to the highest per capita health care costs, the highest mental and emotional barriers to a sense of shared, mutual responsibility. . . .

First of all, let me declare my generic belief of many years—that managed care is better than unmanaged care! . . . Community organization can result in a more efficient, more equitable health system with better outcomes. . . . With the future constraints of finite resource allocation, community health care planning and budgeting will have strong appeal. It is the usual pattern in other advanced nations.

Since Dr. Saward gave that seminal speech, events have borne him out with chilling precision. In the *Portland Oregonian* for April 23, 1991, appeared this news item:

The United States spent a larger share of its gross national product on health care in 1990 than in any year in history, according to preliminary figures released in the new issue of the journal *Health Affairs*.

According to the report, spending on health came to 12.2 percent of the GNP in 1990, or $671 billion, up from 11.6 percent—$604 billion—in 1989. This increase is three times greater than the average annual increase of the past thirty years.

Analysts for the Office of National Health Statistics, who prepared the report, attributed the rise to the continued increase in medical spending coupled with slowing of the economy, which made health command a larger share of the GNP than before.

"Growth in health expenditures has increased faster than the GNP in all but three years since 1960," said Louis W. Sullivan, Health and Human Services secretary.

So health care costs are now absorbing nearly one-eighth of the GNP, and that barely two years after Dr. Saward spoke, when those costs were slightly more than one-ninth of the GNP. That leaves eight years until the costs absorb one-seventh of the GNP, if his predictions prove to be accurate.

But it may be worse than that. Increasingly, these are costs the nation can no longer afford. Consider these other large-type headlines from the same newspaper over a period of less than two years:

## WASTING AWAY

HEALTH-CARE COSTS SOARING, BUT 25% OF MONEY IS WASTED

Evidence is now overwhelming that at least 25% of the money Americans spend on health care is wasted. And all those wasted billions would be more than enough to fill the gaps and provide all the immediate and long-term care our people need.

—Joseph A. Califano, Jr., secretary of Health, Education and Welfare from 1977 to 1979.

MEDICARE REFORM WOULD CUT COSTS, IMPROVE CARE

The U.S. lags far behind other industrialized countries in some basic health indices, including average life expectancy.

—Dr. Louis Sullivan, secretary of Health and Human Services.

ECONOMICS OF HEALTH, HIGHER EDUCATION TRIGGER BACKLASH

Health and higher education are on the public griddle, and though the two industries have little in common, their plight has the same origin—a never-never land system of economics that's generating a backlash among customers.

—Daniel S. Greenberg, editor and publisher of the *Science and Government Report.*

AIDE SAYS HEALTH COSTS SINKING U.S. FISCAL SHIP
Runaway health costs are jeopardizing the nation's long-term economic stability and sinking the federal government into deeper debt, Bush administration budget director Richard G. Darman told Congress April 16 [1991].
Health spending will overtake Social Security as the biggest item in the federal budget by the end of the century, according to Darman.
    —Z. A. Zaldivar, Knight-Ridder News Service

There is no way in which a problem of this magnitude can be resolved as a single stand-alone issue. And it's not simply a matter for legislation, or for administration consideration and action, or even for reform in the health care industry itself. This economic monster has been growing incrementally for the past fifty years, and it will be resolved over time only by deliberate, persistent, rational scrutiny in all public forums, followed by courageous and determined action at all levels.

The root of the problem lies in the way our health care system has developed. The process was explained in this way by Drs. David U. Himmelstein and Steffie Woolhandler in the *Annals of Internal Medicine* in 1988:

> Over the past century medical care has evolved from a small cottage industry, through a period of rapid expansion as a charitable public service, to an enormously profitable and increasingly private business. Medicine has become one of the largest industries in the United States, and economics now competes with science and humanitarian concerns in shaping the future of medical care. . . . We argue that the growth of prospective payment (such as health insurance plans administered through HMOs) can be traced to an implicit compromise between cost-conscious corporate purchasers of care and corporate health providers struggling to expand profitability and assert control of medicine.

The writers point out that the application of industrial (i.e., mass production) methods in health care has resulted in bigger

17

and better-equipped hospitals, organization of larger and more versatile clinics to serve larger numbers of patients, and investment of capital to buy the increasingly costly machines used in high-tech diagnostic and treatment procedures. After developing this thesis in detail, the authors conclude:

> A reorientation of policy will require an alternative coalition of forces capable of resisting the imperatives of pecuniary interests. Physicians together with other health care workers and our patients may provide such a force.

In my opinion, the writers have presented a cogent analysis of the economic trends in health care, involving the distortions that have grown largely from competitive factors. But their one-sentence concluding proposal is clearly inadequate. Physicians, health care workers, and patients, without a countervailing plan and powerful incentives of their own, can scarcely stem the strong-running tide of inflating costs. It is my intention simply to point in some promising directions, like isolated weather vanes in the general storm, and to suggest some concrete activities that could start the ball rolling without any initial legislation, funding allocation, or new agencies. There must be at least as much pressure from below as from above if the tide is to be not merely halted, but rolled back to more rational levels before it inundates even more of our landscape.

From January 1989 until the spring of 1990, I had spent more than a year researching the problem of overmedication and mismedication of seniors. When I discovered that I had covered all the principal bases, I realized that there was little information telling a formerly prescription-drug-dependent person like myself what I could, or should, have done to prevent this from happening. It then occurred to me that most of the professionals I had talked to, each an expert in some phase of the problem, did not know or had not discussed their own experiences with other members of the group. I believed it would be useful if I were to assemble some of them in a symposium setting and see if some kind of consensus or creative synthesis would occur.

So, with the cooperation of Jean Dunlop, staff supervisor of the Alcohol and Chemistry Dependency Program for Older Adults at St. Vincent Hospital in Portland, I organized such a meeting, at which the faculty of nine presented their experiences and perspectives. The one thing that came out of the meeting, which had not been articulated beforehand, was that problems such as overmedication have to be handled by teams of caregivers, professionals, and volunteers cooperating to meet all the needs of elderly patients—emotional, spiritual, domestic, and financial—as well as the purely physical and medical.

I then realized that the focus of my research would have to change if I were to get to the heart of the problem. I could see that overmedication and mismedication were only one aspect of a larger health care problem that, as Dr. Saward pointed out, threatens the foundations of our national economy and the fabric of society. The focus of my research had to change because I realized that our models of health care have to change.

I don't have the resources, the time, or the scholarship to attempt a one-man synthesis of this magnitude. But I have learned enough to have some confidence in pointing out a route along which efforts should be directed, and to suggest the philosophical framework on which the final structure can be built.

I started by developing further the concept of health-care teams as it applies to the elderly. This concept will be explored in the remainder of Part I.

The other three segments of the book will deal with changes I think will be needed in the administration of health care itself, with ways in which healing modalities can be blended into a more effective program, and with the driving force behind the present effort—the need for greater individual responsibility and a dedication to ethical and spiritual direction in the whole enterprise.

# 3. Principles of Team Care

Are there existing models of successful health care teams serving the elderly? Are there firm principles on which the team programs are built? Certainly. Principles first, then models; then some suggestions about organization and leadership.

The principles, really, are more a statement of the rationale for the teams than the kind of axioms and laws one studies in geometry and physics. There's nothing very hard and fast about this; a lot of it is common sense, but a little guidance may be useful in getting into the problem.

1. You have to go into the homes where the elderly are if you are going to find them and give them any kind of help. The elderly seldom come into social service agencies by themselves. Their doctors see them, but seldom in the context of anything more than "the symptom of the day." It's true that caregivers will often make the first contact, but even so, home visitation is recommended as the way to get a first-hand "feel" for the problem. Just the eyeball evidence of the household surroundings will tell the experienced evaluator a lot about a patient. The conversation will be more relaxed, the answers more freely given, confidence more quickly established, and the relationship more nearly friend-to-friend than in a doctor's office or agency headquarters. And how do you find these elderly? More about that later.

2. In every care program, large or small, some kind of initial assessment or evaluation is a must if the care team is to be properly organized and care priorities set. In nearly all cases, this should be done by an experienced person, as patients will not otherwise volunteer sufficient information, and inexperienced people may not be persistent enough to make sure key questions are answered. A well-organized team will use a well-organized questionnaire and will make sure it is completely filled out.

3. There are often important non-medical issues that must be addressed. Dr. Phyllis McGraw, speaking at my symposium on medication, said she had learned through her studies at the University of Southern California that there is a need for specific programs to address the needs of older adults and the cultural issues older adults have. Some of the issues of older people are multiple and irretrievable losses, which are different from the losses younger people might have, she said, pointing out that younger people can often regain the losses they experience, but when the older people lose others from their own families or from among their friends, it is through death.

"And they may lose their actual identity, because during their working years they were always identified through their careers, especially men," she concluded. "Those issues —losses of various kinds including health—apply to all older people. This is inevitable as we get older."

4. I have concluded that one needn't wait for the perfect program to come along, but should get something started with a few key volunteers and minimal staff direction. Anything is better than nothing. People who are hurting want help on their time, not yours. Waiting for a grant from a foundation— or for a bill to get through Congress—may be like waiting for a gold-plated padlock for the barn door while thieves are making off with horses, colts, hay, oats, and tack.

5. Individuals and teams should tap into whatever educational resources are available. The county agencies dealing with needs of the aging, as well as churches, health organizations, and support groups, have a wealth of books and pamphlets

describing chronic ills of the elderly as well as common emotional and psychological disturbances. National headquarters of such organizations, whose addresses are included in the literature, will supply more information on request. Often the problem is to sift out what is useful and what is not, as well as to ask a doctor or well-informed friend whether it applies to a particular case. The only caution is that for conditions such as diabetes, one's doctor should be the final authority as to treatment.

6. Continuity of care and follow-up are always important, and never more so than when dealing with homebound patients. Minutes and hours are paramount to these lonely people, and to let days go by without a look-see or telephone check can be very harmful to the relationship.

7. There may be problems of allocation of resources if there aren't enough to go around. I've been told that 5 percent of the elderly patients get 85 percent of the resources, while the other 95 percent get only 15 percent, so you can see where the pressures for funds and technological equipment come from. It has been pointed out, however, that this is what we should expect—those who are chronically ill or hospitalized are the ones who get the expensive care, while those who are relatively healthy may require little in the way of resources. And indeed, this is the way insurance works—and that includes Medicare. However, you don't have to be smart to see that if we could keep more people healthy longer (or if they could keep themselves healthier!), we would save money and resources all the way around. The local application of this is that health care agencies might have to enforce some kind of triage, such as "first to the neediest." Otherwise, one of three things may happen: the wealthiest or most aggressive—or best insured—might monopolize the available goods and services; in some situations, the indigent frail elderly might be the only ones who qualify for help; or both the first and third groups might be taken care of, while the traditional loser—the self-supporting middle-income taxpayer—might wind up with little or no help. Care managers have to be alert to that kind of situation.

8. Planning ahead is a hot topic in senior care circles, according to Joan Greathouse, manager of senior programs for Group Health Cooperative of Puget Sound. She says this involves both training and information, and covers such subjects as wills, durable powers of attorney, advance directions, health care plans, financial plans, housing, and long-term care. The recognition of this need is just beginning and older adults are interested in learning more about these subjects.

9. All who work with elders agree that programs must be specially geared to elders' needs, or else the elders may be pushed to one side when brigaded with younger and more energetic participants. And some programs must be gender-specific—that is, designed for men only or women only. This may seem to be discriminatory, but if in fact a support group attracts seventeen men and only one woman, or twenty women and two men (as often happens), those in the minority often drop out and receive no service at all.

10. Workers must be alert to signs of neglect or abuse of their clients. Jacque Wallace, former director of a residential program for women alcoholics in Bothell, Washington, says that 95 percent of chemically dependent women have been incested, molested, or raped, and 100 percent have been abused. This indicates the extent of the emotional and psychological problems that may have to be confronted by anyone trying to help a woman who comes to a program by this route.

11. A large number of cases, probably a majority, will come in through the intervention of a third party—a family member, church worker, or doctor who recognizes that the individual has passed the bounds of normal self-help or routinely available support. Actually persuading the client or patient to seek or accept help often has to be done by a professional, in which case a family member will have to enlist such help to get things started. Jacque Wallace, quoted above, says that formal intervention is the ultimate act of love. It is far more likely to happen in the later stages of a dependency, or when a crisis occurs, so the intervener is seldom guilty of haste in this respect.

12. Elders frequently suffer from some degree of memory loss, and team members must keep this in mind in setting up care plans and schedules. Very often, there is no caregiver present to see that programs are followed.

13. Some form of stress control is often required. Medication can help in some cases, but may not be appropriate if clients have learned to deal with their own mental and emotional responses to stressors. If they have not learned this, the team should address this lack as a top priority.

14. Confidence-building is critical. Seniors cannot be rushed into decisions and relationships. People working with them should be respectful and attentive, making sure the older person understands what is being said and agrees with any decisions reached.

15. Where there are psychological problems, at least one team member must be competent to detect and act upon any signals that warn of suicide or self-damage by the patient.

16. Finally, elders should be encouraged at every step to question what is being done to or for them, and to reach out for help if something is bothering them. *This will not work* unless time is available for conversation and reflection. Dorothy Sullivan, a retired nurse with experience in senior care, says she would sometimes engage in talks with her older hospital patients, who would occasionally start to cry and spill out the things that were actually bothering them. This would lead to changes in their treatment, and start the true healing process. But Dorothy would be criticized by doctors and other nurses for "spending too much time with the patient"!

Other important considerations are:

Team models based mainly on volunteer effort have two advantages: seniors helping seniors are often more effective than younger persons; and volunteers can play a critical role in reducing health care costs. Not only are their services free in most cases, but they may be uniquely qualified to serve as team leaders or peer counselors. The *VIEWS* program in Portland, which I'll describe later, is based almost entirely on volunteer effort, with a paid staff of only three persons keeping the whole program afloat.

Very often, patients who are energetic and well informed are able to get their own teams going. For them, this book may offer some encouragement and ideas, because they are not alone. With perhaps rare exceptions, every county in the nation has some form of social services that include a senior arm, and various kinds of help are available directly or by reference, often without cost. Dr. Bernie Siegel, in his book *Love, Medicine and Miracles*, calls these self-starters "exceptional patients." These are the patients, he says, who have the courage to love and the courage to work with their doctors to participate in and influence their own recovery. Their judgments and instincts are often superior to those of others, even professionals, because no one else can know them as well as they know themselves.

Teams may not at first see a need for residential care facilities for their clients, but such facilities may be down the road for many. Oregon is a leader among states in adopting policies to keep people in their own homes and communities wherever and as long as possible. But access to adult foster homes, assisted-living facilities, skilled nursing homes, and long-term care institutions should be catalogued and evaluated in advance. In some cases, this will include a hospice house environment for clearly terminal cases.

The elderly are often unsophisticated about medical matters and inclined to rely on their doctors for any help they need. Doctors say, "Most of my patients aren't looking for anything special—they just want to be treated." And as long as the patients themselves are comfortable and functional with the pills and diets they have, they seldom look further. They may become bewildered if they have to research new medications, as when they try to read the package inserts that come with prescription drugs (if the type isn't too small for *anyone* to read).

# 4. Functions of the Team

The points enumerated above summarize the rationale for a team approach to health care for the elderly. The key points are that older persons differ in their needs for care, both because of mounting physical problems and because of pressures caused by losses, retirement, end-of-life concerns, and other emotional and spiritual issues.

In thinking about developing a team for any particular situation, we must consider four aspects: its function; its composition; its finance; and its leadership. These aspects are so tightly interlocked that it is hard to write about one without writing about all, but I shall consider them separately to keep the picture clear. I think readers will be able to make their own connections and comparisons, meanwhile having handy checklists for testing the suitability of any particular model.

The entire range of functions is designed in every case to do one thing: to support the elderly clients in living the most satisfactory lives possible, considering their physical condition, home environments, and available resources. Some clients may need support in only one area, such as transportation to and from doctors' offices. Others may require the whole gamut of support services. The well-designed team will be able to accommodate all, with minimum lost time or duplication or waste of resources.

If you will bear with one more numbered list, I'll suggest the following as the functions most often needed:

1. Primary care from a qualified medical doctor, and access to specialists as required.
2. Support from other health care professionals such as nurses, therapists, and psychologists.
3. Provision for adequate and healthful diets and food supplies.
4. Monitoring and instruction concerning medication.
5. Transportation to appointments, senior centers, recreational activities, visits and short trips, and so on.
6. Help with paying bills, keeping checkbooks in balance, and handling other money matters.
7. Help with wills, dealing with real and personal property, and other legal concerns.
8. Personal counsel and treatment as needed to meet emotional and relational needs.
9. Help with hospitalization and all the stressful complications involved.
10. Help with health insurance and claims.
11. Home cleaning and maintenance and yard work as necessary.
12. Conservation of personal effects, and making disposition as desired by the patient.
13. Arranging for medical equipment during illnesses and convalescence.
14. Answering inquiries and correspondence.
15. Looking ahead to final arrangements in the event of death, and assuring patients that their wishes will be complied with.
16. Attention to social support and contact with others.
17. Respite for caregivers, usually a spouse or relative. Without occasional relief, full-time caregivers often become primary patients themselves.
18. Personal counseling. Just as people have doctors and lawyers, they need one person to give sound, sympathetic but objective advice on a wide range of subjects.

19. Frequent, perhaps daily contact to assure the team that the patient is safe and alert.
20. Personal care—baths, hair care, getting dressed, and so on.
21. Taking care of the wardrobe—laundry and dry cleaning, replacing worn items.

The list may have to be shortened or lengthened depending on the patient, but team leaders should have complete freedom to do this within limits of time, energy, and money.

I have said before, and I repeat, that no two patients are alike; hence the composition of the health care team may vary from case to case. At one extreme is the loving, competent, committed caregiver who provides everything but skilled medical care for the patient. At the other is the team that has to do everything for the ailing, elderly person who lives alone and suffers from fears and crushing emotional problems in addition to physical ills. And everything in between.

# 5. Organization of the Team

What is a team, as envisioned by this book? How is it organized, who are its members, and how is it led? What gives it its authority, or, more important, its acceptance or cachet? How is it kept together, and how is its success measured? How does it acquire its patients, and who decides when its services are no longer needed?

The first of these questions—how the team is organized and led—can be answered rather easily, and will be dealt with here. The other questions—authority, acceptance, and evaluation of results—are much more qualitative and subject to argument, and so will be considered when we describe existing models of team operation at the end of this section.

In looking at how a team is organized—or more basic, how it gets started in the first place—I like to use the analogy of a fungal spore in a petri dish. In the right environment, the fungus will thrive and spread, and eventually will take over the whole laboratory, making other considerations moot.

The team movement should be like this. You don't start with legislation or by petitioning the American Medical Association or major drug companies for help. If you can find all or some of the functions already established and available through a county health department or other agency, so much the better. But you don't have to wait for this or for someone else to tell you what to do. You start by just doing it, with in-home, hands-on, trial-and-error effort by yourself and anyone else whose help you can enlist; through love, determination, common sense, improvisation, courage, daring, negotiation, communication, public appeals, or any other ethical means. The effort may involve you as a patient or caregiver, and may include other elderly people themselves.

The team organizer, the team leader, the coordinator, and the evaluator may be the same person, or, in impersonal agencies handling a number of cases simultaneously, it may be several people working together. Whatever the organizational diagram, the role of leader or leaders should be clearly understood by everyone on the team.

The obvious candidates for leadership in many cases are the patient or the family doctor. Whatever their status in the team pecking order, they're going to be important members of the team, and both may have the veto power over any decision regarding the patient's physical health. The patient, given enough energy, knowledge, and desire, is the ideal leader; other members of the team, however, must be prepared to support the patient in his (her) decisions, and to take over the decision-making authority when the patient can no longer do so. This question can sink the best team or damage family relationships more easily, perhaps, than any other, if it is not settled in advance while the patient is still in full possession of his (her) faculties.

Ask any doctor or lawyer about cases in which elderly clients lay helplessly in bed within a few weeks, days, or hours of death while sons and daughters, nieces and nephews, and others in the extended family argue in an adjoining room over any one of a thousand details that should have been settled by the patient long before. If the patient doesn't have the foresight to do this, the doctor, lawyer, or prospective executor should force the issue while there is time, before the arguments and disruptions occur. The wishes of the principal will then be in writing and enforceable upon all.

Most doctors will say they should be the team leaders, but when questioned, they concede that their writ extends only to the physical health of the patient. They are, of course, involved in life-extension matters in terminal cases, and these may be resolved by living wills or durable powers of attorney. Lacking one or both of these, the team leader (if not the doctor) should continue to rely on the family physician as the authority in medical decisions, reserving the right to a second opinion. No other member of the team should presume to make an end run around these two, unless he is prepared for messy litigation.

Regardless of their own opinions, however, doctors are not necessarily the first or even second choices for team leadership. This will probably go by default to a spouse or to adult sons or daughters when one of these is available and willing to assume the responsibility. The caveat here is that the part should be assumed willingly, and anyone who feels himself or herself to be truly unqualified should have the option of declining. In this case, the job of leader may devolve on a person outside the family, such as a caregiver, organization, or community agency.

Once past patients, doctors, spouses, family members, and primary caregivers, the field is wide open to other candidates. Among types who can and do provide leadership in caring for the elderly are social workers, nurses of several types, counselors, pastors or other church workers, close friends and neighbors, lawyers, or perhaps others with a special interest. The team leaders are usually volunteers in the sense that they are not paid just for heading the team; on the other hand, an average volunteer performing routine services such as housework or delivering hot meals will not often be qualified or interested in being a team leader. There's just too much to do and to think about. But these are some obvious qualifications:

- The leader should be free to visit patients in their homes fairly often, to keep close track of patient condition and changing needs.
- The leader should have a good knowledge of available facilities and the kinds of support the patient will need as his (her) condition deteriorates.
- The leader should be able to make decisions solely on the basis of what is best for the patient, without showing favor or providing an economic benefit to any supplier or other interest.

31

❡ The leader should be able to make choices that will balance conservation of the patient's resources with willingness to obtain equipment and services such as lift chairs or massages that will truly benefit the patient.

❡ The leader should have enough free time to make sure the patient's interest is always served, that decisions are not neglected or postponed, that other team members are kept informed of progress, and that family members are involved in decisions and discussions.

Above all, the team leader must have the kind of commitment to the patient that will ensure acceptance and a continuing warm relationship free of stress and worry on the patient's part.

You can see from this why the leadership role is the key to success of the team operation. Without clear and firm guidance from the top, the other members of the team will have a hard time reaching their goals.

Once the initial question of leadership is settled—and it will usually be settled immediately when the right person steps into the role—the makeup of the remainder of the team falls readily into place. There are two types of teams: the ad hoc team that comes together at one time and place to serve one patient, and the "top-down" team that has been organized by experiment and experience to serve a number of patients with similar characteristics including geographic location, type of illness, degree of self-sufficiency, financial status, and so on. Most teams that come about because of the need of one patient in one place at one time are of the first type: most teams that serve many elderly, single patients within a small area are of the second type.

How many team members there are and what qualifications are needed will depend on the kinds of illnesses and conditions involved. The ad hoc teams will be organized through a common-sense approach, bringing in the minimum number of skills and services required; the agencies or institutional teams will pull their members together to meet the perceived needs of a group of patients—for example, the frail indigent elderly in a minority population within a neighborhood or metropolitan district.

The same skill categories will have to be considered for team membership as those we mentioned for team leadership, from social workers and nurses to lawyers. There must be a few additions, however. One of these is the specialist, a doctor by referral, who will join the team because he has been called by the primary care physician to consult or treat a patient with a particular illness. The specialist will be a key member of the team for that patient only. It is not likely that the specialist will or could be the team leader.

Another case is that of the pharmacist. He may play an important role in situations involving continuing medication. He should counsel the doctor and patient about drug dosages, timing, interactions, and similar matters. He should not be overlooked if emergencies occur in which the patient's prescriptions play a part. Team leaders should talk to patients about their drugs and who supplies the drugs, and then look to that pharmacist to be a player on the team, especially if he is willing to be contacted on nights and weekends, when emergencies often arise.

When we talk about team models a bit farther on, we'll also see that one more element is needed—the evaluator, who makes the first assessment of the patient to determine what needs to be done, and who may not be needed further except for periodic up-dating. Sometimes the team leader is the evaluator if he (she) has the history of the case in hand and the technical competence to make an assessment. In most programs, these evaluators get special training to make sure they can do the job with accuracy and sensitivity.

Sometimes the family doctor gets the process started by calling a relative or a care agency and suggesting that something more needs to be done for a patient than treatment for physical ills. The evaluator may be a psychologist or counselor if the primary problem is one of emotional stress or mental health. It may be a person who is trained as evaluator by a social service agency. Whoever does it or however it's done, the evaluation is used to determine what needs to be done and who is going to do it.

A different category of team members are those who give second-echelon service. These are people, paid or volunteer, who do the housekeeping, the laundry, the yard work, the maintenance and repair, and who give the physical attention the patient needs to remain at home instead of being in an institution. I know a woman of eighty-one who lives in a large house by herself, and acts as her own team leader. She is not really ill, just lacking the strength and energy to do many of the chores she has always handled herself. She keeps a chart on the wall over her telephone; this shows days of the week across the top, and the names of friends, volunteers, and handymen down the side who have agreed to take care of certain duties for her. Some are paid and some are not. She fills the spaces on the chart with check marks to show who is doing what. This has been working well so far, so the woman can be in complete control of the situation without having to do many of the things needed for pleasant living. Everyone should be as well organized as she is!

There's another type of volunteer who may hold the key to a new and better model of health care team. This person is the peer counselor, another elderly man or woman whose age, interests, and outlook parallel those of the patient at many points. The peer counselor provides many of the critical skills not often available from other team members. In addition to the attributes of leadership cited earlier, the peer counselor should provide a frequently missing element—the ability to reassure the patient concerning existing situations or plans, plus the ability to convince the patient that certain courses of action should be pursued.

A common and very important example is the need to convince a patient that he (she) should seek help for a mental problem. Seniors are naturally reluctant to do this, often denying that a need exists. Peer counselors are uniquely positioned to do this persuading, as they have the patient's confidence and respect, can help him deal with his fears, and can provide the information about the treatment that will make it attractive to the patient.

The qualifications and duties of peer counselors will be explained in our discussion of existing team models a bit later.

Many other types of professionals and health organizations may become involved in team operations from time to time.

Here's a partial list:

❧ Senior service and education departments of hospitals and health maintenance organizations (HMOs);
❧ Rehabilitation programs of many kinds, from drug and alcohol centers to physical therapy and convalescent facilities;
❧ Various medical support people such as geriatric mental health specialists;
❧ Equipment lending or rental services operated by clubs and hospitals;
❧ Meals on Wheels, in-home visitation services, volunteer secretaries, etc.

I know a lot of readers may be thinking, "All this team business may be very fine, but isn't it just going to be an added expense? How are we going to pay for it? Is it covered by Medicare?"

Certainly the question of finance has to be addressed. Some of the answers are suggested in the preceding text. Others are implied by the nature of the team operations I have described. And still others will have to be studied and figured out within the framework of existing facilities and new programs that may be needed. I think the following trends will be established if the suggested steps are taken:

1. Many new human resources, principally senior volunteers, will be recruited at very little or no additional cost;
2. The kinds of preventive medicine practiced and the models of education and healing agencies to be discussed in Part III will result in a gradual easing of pressures on Medicare and a lessening need for services to the elderly by the medical establishment;
3. An increase in the numbers of motivated paraprofessionals in a number of fields, such as community mental health service, will, in effect, trade high-cost medical doctors' hours for lower-cost maintenance hours.
4. More patient involvement in treatment plans and preventive medicine services, more patient education, and more prepara-

tion of prospective retirees for the problems that come with retirement will have the same effect—cutting health care costs.

5. Continuing pressure will be exerted on Medicare to expand coverage in areas of health-impacting stresses, while health agencies adopt a carrot-and-stick approach to lowering the rates of patient-controllable illnesses—those associated with smoking, alcohol, obesity, sedentary lifestyles, poor habits of rest and sleep, and so on.

This list could be expanded, but I think it suggests some avenues for money-saving developments.

The need will continue for grants from federal, state, and local governments, from foundations and corporations, and for the loans of social scientists and student researchers to enable promising new programs for senior health to be carried out. The challenge is to identify the programs that are successful and to make sure they are continued by somebody, in some form, after the present grant money runs out. You can always expect the paid staff to want their own sources of income to be continued. But acknowledging that, my observation is that money is so hard to get and most of the programs are doing so much good with such limited resources, that the push for more and better programs should generally be supported.

I haven't meant to research the money question exhaustively, as that is distinct from the question of better ways of providing health care for the elderly. But I think it's fair to say that questions of financing will not prevent a start in many of the proposed directions.

It is difficult to specify how and when care teams can or should be organized, because the need frequently exists before anyone realizes that the resources already in place—the caregivers and support people—are inadequate to the task, whether in numbers, skills, or both. So what should happen is that the responsible party or parties, a spouse, or neighbor, or doctor, should take the first step simply by deciding that an organization is needed, and someone should lead it. Most often, the party making that decision will be the *de facto* team leader, at least initially.

Then the people already in support of the ailing party are contacted, notified of the roles they are playing or expected to play, and asked to continue or to coordinate certain activities with other designated members of the team. A lot of this is plain common sense; but it is important that all this is *communicated*, so that each player becomes aware of his or her own specific role, and how it dovetails with the roles of all the other players. Then, as team members are added, the meshing and coordination is updated and the functioning kept smooth and effective as time moves along. All this, of course, with the full knowledge and approval of the client being served, assuming the necessary degree of "savvy" on his or her part.

# 6. The Ad Hoc Team

Where are some of these elder-care teams already up and functioning successfully? At the bottom of the ladder is the ad hoc team put together by one or a few caregivers—spouses and adult children—to take care of an aging person who lacks the skill and energy to do this for himself (herself). My friend Bob, who lives in a nearby town of about 30,000, is an example of this. He and his wife were living alone, in the house they had bought fifty years earlier, the house in which they had raised their three children, and which was still filled with the familiar furnishings and implements of a lifetime.

About five years ago, Bob's wife, Mildred, slipped and fell on a smooth concrete floor while cleaning up after a church dinner. She apparently suffered only a bruised hip and shoulder, no broken bones or other injury. She said it was an accident; she hadn't been dizzy and had had no system of illness.

As time went on, she developed a tremor in her hands that made it difficult to hold things or do work with either hand. Within a few weeks, her doctor diagnosed Parkinsonism and prescribed a medication to provide the dopamine her brain apparently lacked. She showed temporary improvement, but then her condition continued to worsen.

Bob took up the slack as Mildred became progressively less able to do her usual chores. He did the shopping and more and more of the cooking and housework. One by one, Mildred was compelled to give up her duties. Doing the laundry, putting away linens and clothes, making and changing beds, vacuuming and dusting—pretty soon, Bob was doing it all. Yard work, which had never been Bob's forte, was almost totally neglected, except for an occasional mowing. Plants began to dry up because they were not watered.

And soon Mildred's mental faculties began changing. She could no longer do things for herself, but she could still worry about them and charge Bob with seeing that they were done. He had always tried to please Mildred in every way, but now he had to answer increasing demands from her while doing all the unaccustomed tasks himself.

The situation soon reached a point at which Bob knew he had to reach out for help, or suffer some kind of collapse himself. The first step in team-building (although Bob didn't think of it that way) was to hire a woman to come in and do the laundry and cleaning once a week. As Mildred's condition worsened, Bob was able to find a young woman of about twenty to come in three mornings a week and be a companion to Mildred while he went shopping or did a few things on his own.

Over the next six months, many changes occurred as Mildred continued to lose ground. A local public health nurse was called upon to visit Mildred regularly to check on her condition and monitor her medication. Women from the church would bring in casseroles or salads from time to time. Mildred's physician took to dropping in once or twice a week, on his way to or from hospital rounds, just to check in person.

Poor Bob! Because Mildred was no longer ambulatory, a wheelchair had to be rented; and because she couldn't climb stairs, Bob had to buy a mechanical lift for about $1,500 and have it installed in place of the stairs between the back porch and the driveway.

The wheelchair was too wide for the bathroom door, so a new door was cut in the wall between the bathroom and hallway. Mildred grew weaker and weaker. She could no longer speak. She could not prevent strange movements of her arms, frequently raising them over her head as she lay in bed.

She was hospitalized twice to stabilize scary symptoms, and finally, on the third trip to the hospital, she died.

The pattern of the illness, and Bob's response to it, are all too familiar. As the primary caregiver, he started from a position of almost total ignorance of Mildred's probable support requirements, and what the local sources of support might be. He had to meet each emergency as it arose, with varying, if not conflicting, counsel from his doctor, his relatives, his neighbors, and associates. There was no single experienced advisor to point out the possible course of Mildred's illness and her potential needs. Nor was there any great amount of coordination between the sources of help Bob called upon. He felt he was alone in shouldering responsibility and making decisions, and this at a time when his beloved wife and life's companion was losing her vitality and will to live.

Bob and Mildred are typical of elderly couples who live by themselves, and who do not face the problem of physical impairment until it happens. Then they meet these problems one day at a time, always taken by surprise when conditions worsen, always starting from scratch when making arrangements for further help and treatment. Many such people hope for miracles that never happen. Within my own experience are several cases in which the elderly invalid, slipping rapidly toward the end, will say, "I'm going to see the doctor again tomorrow. Maybe he will finally be able to tell me what's wrong with me!" I think there's less reason to encourage this attitude than to begin to prepare the patient for dying in an atmosphere of serenity and love.

# 7. The Neighborhood Team

Things don't have to be as they happened to Bob and Mildred. We'll look at some other models in which these typical conditions can be planned for and taken care of in an organized way, by trained volunteers and supporting professionals. One such program is that operated in parts of Multnomah County, Oregon, a large metropolitan area with a wide range of neighborhood and population types. Here is part of what Claire Wart, a registered nurse with nursing home experience, told our drug symposium in Portland in April 1990:

"I have been involved in the Block Nurse Program in Multnomah County, Oregon, the largest city being Portland. Local nurses, certified nurses' aides, and volunteers visit older adults in their community who have requested assistance to manage their health and cope with the issues of aging. The frequency of these visits depends on how serious the need is.

"In the fall of 1990, the Block Nurse program ended as a very successful pilot program so that the best elements could be incorporated into an expanded model serving all of Multnomah County. The new model is called a Multi-Discipline Team (MDT) serving the same target population of at-risk people sixty years of age and older. The team is composed of a social worker, a mental health specialist, and a community health nurse. The MDT has linked Aging Services, mental health agencies, and the Health Division to provide a coordination of services.

"Some of the services offered by both these programs are those of advocacy, monitoring, assessment, and validation treatment. We try to maintain people in their homes as comfortably as possible, for as long as possible, trying to maximize the quality of their lives and their sense of having a meaningful existence.

"We have found that clients are often referred to our program because they have been frequently hospitalized or have used the emergency system inappropriately. Many of these clients are not hospitalized again once there is appropriate intervention, and they may be able to die in their own homes as they wished.

"We have gradually changed our approach from one of being experts telling clients what they should do, to an approach that focuses on choices. We teach clients that they are the best experts on who they are. When they see medical providers, whether nurses, pharmacists, or physicians, they utilize them as resources, and feel good about knowledge they have about themselves, and what works for them.

"The clients are encouraged to learn all they can about themselves, to make choices and to observe how it is affecting them. When people are making plans with you, whether it is your doctor, your nurse, a social worker, mental health specialist, or family member, you'll stand up and say, 'I believe . . . I feel confident . . . ' It doesn't mean you don't consider advice of other people, but that you look at it from your own knowledge and perspective. Clients have responded positively to this approach."

Claire provides several case histories of successful service to clients, of which the following is typical (out of two hundred seen up to the time of our interview):

"Mr. G is a 72-year-old diabetic black male living alone, with rapid mental deterioration. His condition left him vulnerable, and as a result he was financially manipulated by several people. He was not able to cooperate with plans to help him stay independent.

"The MDT began seeing him in June 1990, starting by assessing his needs and arranging for a medical evaluation. The mental health specialist saw him and diagnosed severe dementia. A money manager was found. The protective service worker and RN (nurse) provided ongoing monitoring and established a solid relationship with Mr. G so that when a young woman moved in to care for him, they were able to establish quickly that she was abusing him financially. Eventually, staff people helped the client make a decision to move into adult foster care where he is currently living. The MDT is monitoring the situation."

You don't have to try very hard to see the major difference between Claire's work and the experiences of my friends, Bob and Mildred, described earlier. Claire plays the role of the nurse-counselor who takes charge of the case when she walks in the door. She makes the initial assessment. She decides what needs to be done, and either does it or arranges for it to happen. She gains the trust of her clients and can usually persuade them to get the kinds of help they need. She is a committed caregiver who stays with a case until the need ends. She quiets fears, deals with depression and loneliness, and brings a measure of peace of mind to the frightened, confused oldsters. She gets paid, of course. But the cost to the client and the public is minimal. The proof of this lies in her statement, "Many are not hospitalized again once a nurse becomes involved in their homes."

Nor do you have to try very hard to see the major weaknesses in this model. First, there aren't enough Claire Warts to go around. Without the skills of a trained nurse, this model doesn't work.

Second, this is a funded program of the county—minimally funded, true enough, but still relying on money provided through the political process. It works only in neighborhoods where the clients can pay at least a small part of the freight.

Third, the program is in danger of slipping or stopping whenever the nurse-counselor gets sick, moves away, or quits for any reason. All of these factors would have to be addressed if this model were to be adopted on a broad scale by several jurisdictions. But it's certainly a great model and one that can be reproduced almost anywhere that the leadership and demographic factors are favorable.

# 8. The Composite Sponsored Team

It is tempting to dwell on the previous model, but there are too many more to be examined. Let's explore the work being done by VIEWS (Volunteers Involved for the Emotional Well-Being of Seniors). This is a cooperative effort of four agencies in the Portland metropolitan area, funded by grants from seven local corporations and foundations. The program is administered by the Mt. Hood Community Mental Health Center, with three other agencies, RSVP (Retired Senior Volunteer Program), Project DARE (Drug and Alcohol Resources for the Elderly), and the Oregon State Council of Senior Citizens, involved in delivering services.

To quote briefly from the project's modest folder:

"First, trained peer counselors are paired with older adults undergoing emotional stress. The counselors meet with clients in their homes, discuss their needs and problems, counsel them and seek whatever outside support is indicated.

"Second, practitioners (doctors, etc.) with an interest in working with older adults serve as professional volunteers. They work with peer counselors, consulting with other providers, or serve one older adult client without charge.

"Third, a specialist in chemical dependency joins the VIEWS

team to train the volunteers in responding to problems of alcohol and substance abuse."

It is instructive to listen to Gerry Annand, an ordained minister with a master's degree in counseling, who was one of only three-plus paid staff members of VIEWS at the time of my interview.

"A feeling of shame is an important issue for the elderly, such as those with alcohol or drug problems, whether illegal or prescription drugs. That is why peer support and counseling is such an important tool.

"There are just a huge number of elderly in the metropolitan area that need help. The programs here aren't reaching them. Twenty-five to thirty percent of them have mental health problems, but they don't come in for the alcohol and drug problems even though they might need them. But we don't label them—they're all just clients to us.

"These people respond more positively to small groups than to large—six to ten people are plenty. Transportation is a problem when a client comes into the program. Once we get them sober, they can usually drive themselves. If we can end their depressive isolation they will *want* to get out from their homes more. We try to increase their empowerment. Sometimes we meet in their homes so, in a way, the first meetings come to them. The problem is to get them engaged and attached to other human beings.

"Elders don't want to be lectured to or counseled by younger people. Remember, for young folk, life satisfaction is in the future; for elders it is *now*. The prevalent ageism in this country tells us that elders have no future, but we counter that by showing our clients that their future is *today*.

"Our clients first receive a comprehensive psycho-social evaluation by a geriatric mental health specialist, and are then screened for placement with a peer counselor. These counselors get fifty hours of training within a month. After that they meet for two hours a month, half for continuing education and half peer support.

"I'm impressed with the skills of our volunteers. I have no reservation in saying that our peer counselors can do the job.

"The peer counselors start with one client, and work with that person individually. Then if they have enough time, they may pick up other clients."

The components of the VIEWS program are:

1. Recruitment of peer counselors.
2. Screening of counselors through a comprehensive application and a committee interview.
3. Training of counselors as mentioned above. They commit to nine months of volunteer service. If they are recovered alcoholics themselves, we normally require two years of sobriety before we accept them as counselors.
4. Peer support groups attended by clients led by two specially trained peer counselors. These are usually self-perpetuating, because the members want to stay in touch with their friends.
5. Volunteer professionals who do cross-training of each other and of peer counselors.
6. An evaluation procedure to measure the life satisfaction of clients at the beginning and end of the project.

Annand continued, "We measure success as the continued non-use of alcohol, the non-use of drugs except recommended prescription drugs, and no inappropriate use of prescription drugs."

And he concludes, "Don't underestimate the power of trained volunteers!"

There may be some who question the inclusion of an alcohol-drug treatment program in a discussion of health care teams for the elderly, but I defend it on two grounds: First, it is an excellent model that, with some modification, could be used in almost any community care situation; and second, the proportion of alcohol and drug-dependent elders to the total population is so high that a specialized program is fully justified and worthy of emulation.

# 9. The One-Church Team

My fourth model is highly instructive because of the way it came about. This is the Caring Community for Mature Adults (CCMA), a program of Our Lady of the Lake parish in Lake Oswego, just south of Portland. The program was conceived by Dorothy Sullivan, a member of the parish, and she is its director.

Dorothy obtained her nursing degree in 1972, when she was not quite fifty, and seven years later she earned a bachelor of nursing science degree in community health. She worked on a per diem for a few years as a public health nurse, but was forced to give this up by a serious illness. After she recovered, she was asked to help develop a project called OASIS (Older Adult Senior Services and Intervention System) in the San Fernando region of her archdiocese. She worked full time, with a secretary and half-time social worker. They trained volunteers, and did assessments in the homes of the frail elderly, whose needs were met by linking them with appropriate community services.

Dorothy later moved to Lake Oswego and became a member of Our Lady of the Lake parish. Sensing a need for a program like the one she had served in California, she got her priest's permission to organize one for elderly parishioners needing support for physical or emotional reasons.

Dorothy has since recruited a number of volunteers to perform all the tasks needed in meeting the organization's goals, which are:

- To locate and assist older adults who are frail, lonely, isolated, and in need of services.
- To assist their families and friends in providing for their needs.
- To prevent premature or inappropriate institutionalization.
- To help older adults remain in their homes.
- To affirm the presence, talents, and wisdom of older adults.
- To initiate lifelong wellness programs.
- To provide information and referrals as needed.

With only a small room, a telephone, and minimal office equipment supplied by the parish, Dorothy has developed a written statement of purpose; a form for prospective volunteers; an application for older adults needing assistance; a form to be used in volunteering financial and other support; an assessment form for cataloging the needs of elderly clients; a volunteer's monthly report, and a reassessment form to update client's progress and needs. She has also held a workshop on "How to start a parish program."

The "caring community" envisioned by Dorothy is up and running, with a growing volunteer staff and a cadre of elders being served.

It is hard to spot any defects in Dorothy's program. Because of her background as a paid professional in California, she knows how to organize a project of this kind and put it into operation. I could see no ways in which it departed from any of the principles I have discovered during my investigations. It does seem to depend on Dorothy's continuing direction, ingenuity, and dedication, but I'm sure she has in mind the need to develop staff support from younger volunteers, with an eye to turning over the directorship when she becomes unable to continue. Dorothy is now in her late sixties, but seems to be infused with the energy and stamina of a much younger person as she goes about her new-found career.

Through her organization, she is certainly saving society a ton of money. She will, no doubt, substantially meet the seven-point goals listed previously, thereby improving the quality of life, the health, and positive outlook of those she serves. And anyone with equal dedication and training can do the same thing, anywhere in the country!

# 10. The Hospital Team

Another example of a well-coordinated health care team serving the elderly, more typical of what is available in many communities nationwide, is that of the Senior Health Services of Good Samaritan Hospital in Portland. Pam Wheeler, the director, has been with the agency for the past eight years.

"We began looking at health services for older people about ten years ago," Pam says. "We had the idea that this was a mission that had to be undertaken, serving this important population needing health care. We realized we had to take a different approach from one used with younger people.

"We began by setting up a gerontology program built around a health care team of a physician, a psychologist, and a nurse. We had no social worker on the team at that time. The nurse would go into peoples' homes to see how they functioned, how they could get around and do things for themselves, which is a lot more important than their age. We wanted to help them stay at home longer.

"Sometimes the person's adult children would call us, or the elderly spouse who had become a caregiver.

"As it works now, we have one nurse who takes calls for the gerontology center. The problems are usually some kind of dementia or memory loss, whether Alzheimer's disease or other mental impairment. Then the client is brought in for a clinical workup by a geriatrician, a neuropsychologist, or a neurologist.

If the client needs a physical workup we start with the geriatrician, then a psychologist might track the causes of memory loss. This clinic doesn't do continuing care, but sends clients back to their own doctors and community resources with suggestions for follow-up.

"If primary mental health treatment is needed, however, we do offer this through two geropsychiatrists.

"At the end of the clinical evaluations, we have a family counseling session. We try to put it all together here. We take the time to talk to the clients and their families. All of them really appreciate having this opportunity to have their concerns given a good airing. Incidentally, our mental health clinic is very full.

"We also offer case management through a nurse who gets referrals from the other services I've already mentioned. A staff physician works with her on this. If we can get physicians to identify which clients need this service and which do not, we can step in and give the clients the help they need. Some of their doctors pick up on this and some do not.

"We have a foot clinic that is always full. We do this two times a week. We have a nurse who gives foot massages, cleaning, and trimming of nails. Many older people just stop walking if their feet hurt and we try to prevent this. If they can't walk, they can't take care of themselves.

"We have a linkage with our emergency room and some clients come this way. If an older patient has problems that are non-medical, the ER calls social services and we take over. A good example would be someone who tried to commit suicide by overdosing on pills.

"We also have a health promotion for seniors through our Legacy Health System, which includes five Portland hospitals and the Visiting Nurse Association. We use it to reach seniors throughout the system, and have more than 10,000 enrolled now. We use a newsletter to get health information to seniors, and have a number of special classes for them.

"And we provide long-term care, something few hospital programs do. Our hospital owns the Bishop Morris Care Center which we are converting from intermediate care to a skilled nursing facility, so there is a strong emphasis on rehabilitation.

There is also a unit for Alzheimer's patients. In-home hospice service for terminal patients is through the Visiting Nurses Association.

"One nurse practitioner works with the geriatricians, following up on patients in our Bishop Morris Care Center. We follow about seventy people in this facility, and see them almost daily. When the nursing home staff has a problem they usually call the nurse practitioner rather than the doctor because access is easier. The nurse practitioner is a 'doctor extender' in this respect.

"We are just starting something brand new. We have two geriatrician MDs who are starting a practice in an office adjoining the hospital, focusing on the frail elderly. They want the complex older patient to come to them, mainly because they are geriatric physicians and can refer patients to any other doctor or treatment center they think is best qualified to deal with a particular condition. They can see that patients get help with their finances, insurance, legal matters, and other bothersome problems.

"They will physically be in the same area as our geriatric assessment center, so you might say we'll have 'one-stop shopping' for the elderly needing health care. This is a new direction in applying standard medicine and common sense in handling complex cases.

"The challenge is reimbursement. These cases will take more time. We've developed a hospital-based program because it would be difficult for individual doctors to realize a profit, if in private practice. The hospital will benefit from referrals to and from the doctors, additional lab work, new in-patients and other services we wouldn't have gotten otherwise. We're going to track the sources of revenue and see if this is a self-supporting program."

You will correctly deduce from this rather long description that the hospital program at Good Samaritan is more than a single type of team. Rather it is a grouping of senior health services, well-coordinated so that an older patient with almost any complex of symptoms will receive appropriate care. There may be some gaps, but the organization is sensitive to emerging needs, and is positioned to close those gaps effectively. The one apparent drawback is that the sponsor hospital is constrained to break even financially, if not to show a profit, so any social program that represents a net continuing drain on hospital resources could not be long continued.

Good Samaritan may have a better established and more complete program than most hospitals, but all of the major ones in the Portland area have some type of educational and outreach services for senior citizens. Meridian Park Hospital in Tualatin, for example, has just opened a new health education building that will serve as a focus for more than forty educational and health promotion activities, including support groups for a number of patient categories. The impetus for this movement has several sources: the need for hospitals to broaden revenue-producing services because of cost pressures in traditional areas; the demand by senior advocates, and many seniors themselves, for help in enjoying better health practices; and the growing realization in all fields that the burgeoning population of elders needs new and different kinds of help in improving their health and life satisfaction.

# 11. Group Health Co-op of Puget Sound

The next model I will discuss in detail is the Group Health Cooperative (GHC) of Puget Sound, which is unique among major HMOs in having been launched by the patients themselves, and which is still controlled by the patients through an elected board of directors. GHC went through rocky times in its early years because the medical establishment refused to recognize or cooperate with it, and tried to discredit the doctors with whom it signed contracts. After GHC won its early court battles and proved it could provide good quality health care at moderate prices, however, it not only grew rapidly in Seattle and surrounding areas, but became recognized as a leader in delivering health care to a wide spectrum of patients.

The bold-face type in the policy statement in GHC's 1989 annual report capsulizes the organization's philosophy:

"As a cooperative, we value our system of *consumer governance*. . . . Group Health was a pioneer in *managed health care*. . . . Our system of managed health care nurtures *high quality*. . . . Group Health values *preventive care* and *health promotion*. . . . Integrally tied to health care is *research*."

The 1990 fact sheet for GHC and its affiliate, Group Health Northwest (GHNW), reports a total enrollment of 439,131 participants. Opened in 1947, it is the nation's sixth oldest HMO, and the largest such cooperative. It had estimated revenues for 1989 of $529 million. As of January 1, 1990, it had 8,222 full- and part-time staff members, including 822 physicians and other medical staff, and 1,445 nurses. It is the ninth largest employer in the state of Washington. It also contracts with 1,256 outside physicians to provide services in locations where there is no appropriate GHC staff.

Considering the broad and comprehensive scope of GHC's mix of patient services, its policies with respect to senior enrollees are noteworthy. These policies run on two tracks—one, the direct service to elders in the normal course of doctor-patient relationships, and the other, the heavy weighting of its community services toward the senior population. GHC is one of the few HMOs, for example, that has general practitioners devoting all or a major portion of their practices to senior citizens.

One of these doctors is Charles Wischman. His average patient is seventy-two years old. Unlike most physicians in America today, Dr. Wischman loves taking care of older people. There are one thousand of them on his patient panel—only a little more than half the number served by most of his fellow doctors, but, as he points out, the seniors require considerably more attention than younger people.

He spends a lot of his time talking to his patients. His aim is to find out what they really want him to do for them. He has learned that none of them want to have their lives prolonged artificially when they are no longer independent.

Dr. Wischman doesn't believe the average life span is threescore and ten. He says that if the genetic factor is right, people should live to be 120, then die of old age. He also reports that most of the problems he treats are what he calls "diseases of agriculture" and abundance—those that result from eating too much fat, protein, and simple sugars.

Dr. Wischman frequently brings his message of better health practices to groups of older Group Health members in a speech entitled "Getting the Most Out of Your First 100 Years."

He counsels greater physical activity at every opportunity. Whatever you can do physically, he advises, you should do—plus a little bit more.

"When you sit around, you're gone," he says.

He tries to stay focused on the patient he's seeing at the moment. He feels the doctor should have a long-range relationship with all his clients. He has found that keeping the same patients year after year enables him to spend less time taking histories, doing examinations, and making tests.

"When I know my patients, I can usually tell in a few minutes what is happening with them," he reports. He also says that much of what needs to be done can be accomplished by his patients in their homes. He says he finds that many conditions can be treated with common-sense remedies, without using expensive medicine and surgeries.

Approaching the problem of senior health care from the standpoint of its entire field of operation, GHC has established a Community Services Department that is a clear model of the team approach. Betty Thornton, director of this department, described its activities in a recent interview.

"Our community services are built on the mission of interdisciplinary service, a feature of Group Health for forty years, the first organization to hire public health visiting nurses in the Seattle area. We have a long tradition in that field, as well as issues of health promotion.

"We now have more than 130 paid employees serving more than 9,000 clients annually, from 'womb to tomb.' We have pediatric and newborn services, also rehabilitation and home-health programs, nursing home liaison, home and community volunteer work, and hospice services.

"This is predicated on the idea that the service needs to make the skills of various practitioners available to each patient in the community, and in his home. The old idea of a single visiting nurse is no longer valid, because there are needs for physical therapy, medical social work, and so on.

"Care extends beyond acute care to the ongoing management of chronic cases. We try to maintain maximum independence for our patients, with home and community volunteers linking the patient to the community. Our volunteers provide non-traditional as well as traditional services. There are friendly visits, helping seniors with shopping and housekeeping, and so on. The idea is to establish a friendly relationship with each patient."

The difference between GHC and other organizations, she pointed out, is that it is a complete *system*, not just an assemblage of segments. The parts do not compete with each other, but reinforce each other, and do not shrink from referring a patient to other parts of the organization.

The largest program of her department is home health. In the outside community, the physician is often reluctant to refer a patient to a home health agency, which he may see as competitive. If the home health program works, the patients may not need to see a doctor so frequently.

In Group Health, each part has a specific role. Its doctors, for example, see the home health capability as a valuable extension of their own treatment.

"This can only benefit the patient," Betty says. "Group Health rates these services very highly. Geriatrics is our bread and butter. It is not just sporadic. Those who deal with the elderly are specialists in geriatrics; they *like* it, and the patients like it because they are in control of their own environment."

A case manager is assigned to each case. The physician defines the medical treatment and protocols, but such things as nursing visits, living activities, and so on may be set up by a nurse, a therapist, a social worker, a spiritual counselor, or other individual.

Besides patients, there are other people who need support because of their status as caregivers. In-home volunteers play a critical role in providing respite to caregivers. If caregivers are supported, then the patient may be able to remain at home longer. Other types of general health insurance don't look at this at all, according to Betty.

"Because of our system, we take these needs into account and try to meet them," she says. "We *know* the neighborhood. Volunteers do chores, provide free meals, knit, drive, do telephoning and letter-writing, and so on. Some are trained in aspects of death, dying, and grieving processes. They also help families at critical times."

Beyond the in-home and clinical services to its enrollees, GHC also has these services for seniors, channeled through a senior information line that provides information concerning any service available to seniors, such as:

- A senior resource center with brochures and other printed information on a variety of health-related subjects. The center also provides consultation on income tax preparation, housing options, legal matters, and so on.
- Medicare enrollment and rate information.
- Health coverage by non-Medicare plans.
- Long-term care through the GHC/Aetna Security Care program.
- A wide range of volunteer services opportunities at twelve GHC group locations.
- A center for health promotion classes.
- A "call central" for information on diets and alternative food choices.
- Help at home, including transportation, household service and respite care, assisted living chores, and home safety.
- Short-term skilled nursing or rehabilitation services for homebound GHC clients.
- Nursing home liaison.
- Hospice care for enrollees with life-limiting illnesses, and their families.
- A telephone visit program.

There are additional medical programs such as speech therapy and prescription-by-mail service. Support groups and mental health services are also available.

Overarching all the senior health care programs is GHC's Senior Caucus, an organization of GHC consumers that serves as an advocate for better health care and services for seniors. It provides a forum for discussion of issues affecting seniors, publishes a newsletter, and offers educational programs. It is acknowledged to be highly influential in decisions made by the GHC board in establishing policies and programs for seniors. Any senior member of GHC is welcome to join a chapter and participate in committee activities of the caucus.

In analyzing the services provided by Group Health Cooperative, it is clear that it combines all of the key elements needed for an idealized senior health care team. Its senior enrollees have automatic access to the home service, social support, and medical treatment tailored to their particular needs. The Senior Caucus makes certain that the voice of seniors will be heard by the policy makers in setting standards for the organization. There is a strong commitment to volunteerism, which helps seniors avoid the trap of isolation and inactivity. The cooperative spirit assures a continuing effort to keep down costs while keeping up quality.

The big problem for GHC, as for other HMOs, comes from its very size. The need for decentralization means there are problems of management, communication, and control that lead to the predictable ills of any bureaucracy. The battles between form and substance are never-ending; sometimes the requirement to file reports takes precedence over the contents. But this does not seem to have penetrated to the level of patient care. I can offer this testimony from a friend of fifty-five years' standing, who writes from Seattle:

"My wife and I have been members of Group Health for more than twenty years and are very well satisfied with it. It covers all our medical expenses, hospitalization, and medicines. They have an excellent staff and specialists in almost all disciplines. If they can't handle something in-house, they refer patients to private facilities and pick up the cost."

In mid-1990, Dr. Charles Strother, with whom I spoke some six months later as reported in the prologue to this book, had presented a series of briefing papers to other members of the Group Health Cooperative staff for their consideration and planning purposes. These had to do with ways in which he thought that organization should approach the problem of health services to seniors. These are some of the points he made:

An adequate system of geriatric care must be based on the premise that geriatric patients are not simply "older adults"—they constitute a distinct and unique population.
℘ They undergo significant psychological changes in vision, hearing, perception, memory, and other cognitive functions.

℉ They undergo physiological changes in the ratio of body fat to body weight; in the functioning of liver, kidneys, and bladder; in respiration and circulation.

℉ They are less capable of carrying out the activities of daily living independently.

℉ They tend to live in a much more restricted social environment and to be more dependent on a social support network.

Not only are geriatric patients different, but geriatric medicine differs in many significant ways from general medicine:

℉ It differs in the goal of treatment. In general medicine, the goal is to treat illness; in geriatric medicine, the goal is to maintain function and quality of life and to control pain.

℉ It differs with respect to the conditions to be treated. The medical problems of the older patient are often more chronic, complex, deteriorating, and unavoidably terminal.

℉ It differs with respect to the facilities required for care. The conventional structure and composition of the primary care staff must be different; hospital beds must be supplemented by facilities for sub-acute, home, and custodial care.

℉ The diagnostic interview differs in that it must assess the auditory, visual, cognitive, and memory capabilities of the patient and must obtain a more comprehensive picture of the patient's physical and social environments.

℉ Treatment planning differs in that it must take into consideration the patient's physical and cognitive limitations; his idiosyncratic responses to drugs; and the availability of a support network and of placement facilities.

A system designed to meet the unique needs of the geriatric population should be based on three fundamental principles:

• **Comprehensiveness.** The health problems of the elderly are so often complex, so often interrelated with the physical and social environments in which they live, and so often affected by their mental health, that the diagnostic process must be much more comprehensive than that required by younger patients with uncomplicated acute complaints. The planning of care must address the multiplicity of the patients' problems.

• **Continuity.** General medicine is primarily concerned with discrete episodes of illness. The responsibility for initiating treatment for different episodes rests primarily with the patient. Geriatric conditions are characteristically chronic and progressive, requiring more initiative on the part of providers to maintain continuity of care.

• **Coordination.** The treatment resources required for geriatric medicine are numerous and involve individuals and agencies other than those provided by the acute care delivery system. This makes essential the task of a coordinator who can assure that the patient does not fall into the gaps between services.

In another paper, Dr. Strother outlined what he thought a model care program, administered by an agency such as Group Health Cooperative, would look like. In light of differences in geriatric care mentioned above, he thought that aspects of the new model should include the following:

❧ Maintenance of health and prevention of illness.
❧ Office care, including acute and intermediate care.
❧ Home care, which includes ramifications other than medical.
❧ Community care.
❧ Long-term care, including nursing home and hospice care.

His strategy for planning would cover the following steps:

❧ Identifying patient needs.
❧ Determining resources required to meet those needs, to include clinical personnel, support, facilities, and funds.
❧ Meeting patient obstacles, such as physical limitations, cognitive and emotional problems, and expectations of cure.
❧ Financial objectives.

The implementation phase would proceed through the following steps:

❧ Determining patient needs; analyzing the needs of a representative sample of patients.
❧ Determining necessary resources; analyzing what resources would be required to meet the needs of the sample of patients.

❡ Developing policies and procedures, based on the program's experience and that of other organizations, as well as multi-disciplinary case studies.

❡ Developing strategies to overcome obstacles to implementation, including obstacles presented by patients, professionals, and inadequate funding.

In a cover letter transmitting these briefing papers to me, Dr. Strother said he thought that the approach of most HMOs, including his own, that attempt to modify the present acute care system in various ways is an extremely inefficient way to go. He thinks the model of the Social HMO, which will be described in the next chapter, may be one way. Noting that the problem of funding remains clouded because of the uncertainty of federal funding of health care, he says:

"While I am not yet sufficiently familiar with the experience of the social HMOs to make a considered judgment, my impression is that enough experience has accumulated with this model to make it possible to design and price a first approximation. . . . It may not be easy to persuade people who have been well-satisfied with their previous care that it can no longer meet their needs and that it is worth the difference (in cost). . . ."

So let us introduce our last model, which in many ways represents the farthest point reached so far in official policy regarding specialized care for the elderly—the Social Health Maintenance Organization. Nothing is yet cast in bronze, and some of the most enthusiastic experimenters, like Dr. Strother, are among the most dubious as to what the final outcome will be. The system is in a state of flux, and will depend to a great extent upon directions taken by the federal government and the states in provision for health care at all levels. But Dr. Strother and I agree on this important reservation: The development of a system of geriatric care need not wait on the solution of that problem. Onward and upward!

# 12. The Social/HMO

Dr. Merwyn (Mitch) Greenlick is director of the Kaiser Permanente Center for Health Research in Portland. At the time I interviewed him in August 1990, he was also acting chairman of the Department of Preventive Medicine at Oregon Health Sciences University. Kaiser Permanente is a large health maintenance organization whose Northwest Region, based in Portland, operates hospitals, clinics, laboratories, and support facilities serving much of northwest Oregon and southwest Washington.

Dr. Greenlick was among the first to recognize the need for more specialized medical care for the elderly following the creation of Medicare in the mid-1960s. As the top researcher at Kaiser, he has overseen the creation of what he says is the best health care reference library in the world. At the end of twenty years of operation, he and two co-authors, Donald K. Freeborn and Clyde R. Pope, published *Health Care Research in an HMO*, a 315-page, hard-cover book that is subtitled *Two Decades of Discovery*.

With that background, it is not surprising that Dr. Greenlick was one of the moving spirits in the establishment of the Social HMO project, an effort by Medicare to design and test a program of specialized care for the elderly. Nor is it surprising that the Kaiser organization, with its facilities and expertise in communicating with its members, was selected as one of four test sites in the United States.

Between the time I interviewed Dr. Greenlick and began finalizing this chapter, the Social HMO Consortium published another of its condensed annual reports, this one entitled "The Social/Health Maintenance Organization: The First Five Years." Because the report is both concise and explanatory, I think it will be profitable simply to pass along some of the key information it contains.

The consortium is made up of a coordinating facility, the Bigel Institute for Health Policy at Brandeis University, and four operating centers. Besides Kaiser Permanente in Portland, the others are the SCAN Health Plan at Long Beach, California; the Metropolitan Jewish Geriatric Center in Brooklyn; and Group Health, Inc., and the Ebenezer Society in Minneapolis.

The mission of the consortium is to shed light on critical policy and practice questions about providing community-based, long-term care, including:

- ℥ How to integrate acute, chronic, and informal care to assure continuity and avoid duplication.
- ℥ How to identify Medicare beneficiaries who, formerly independent, have become functionally dependent and mentally unstable.
- ℥ How to define target groups for long-term care and tailor services to their particular needs.
- ℥ How to define affordable long-term care benefits that are compatible with Medicare.

At the end of 1989, enrollment in the plan had exceeded the demonstration target of 16,000 members by several hundred members. The numbers were: Metropolitan Jewish Geriatric Center, 5,078; Kaiser Permanente, 5,414; SCAN Health Plan, 2,819, and Group Health and Ebenezer Society, 3,256.

Medicare beneficiaries and Medicaid recipients voluntarily join the plan, just as they would join other HMOs. Social HMO enrollees must live in the designated service area, be sixty-five years of age or older, and may not have been in an institution within a thirty-day period prior to enrollment. Certain Medicare beneficiaries are excluded because Medicare pays for their care in other special ways. Between 5 and 10 percent of all members per site would be eligible for nursing home admission but are cared for at home.

The Social HMOs finance in-home, long-term care benefits by pooling existing public and private funding, thus making the program budget-neutral to Medicare. For each person who joins, the Health Care Finance Agency (HCFA, which pays Medicare's bills) pays a monthly premium, adjusted by age, sex, and other factors, which is equal to Medicare's expected costs for a similar person in the fee-for-service sector. Each member then pays a monthly premium similar to that of regular Medicare supplements, ranging from zero to $75 at the four sites.

The success of the program is predicated on its ability to deliver both acute and long-term care services on a managed-care basis. Long-term care services are authorized only after assessing each person's eligibility and personal situation. The efficiency of managed care allows the Social HMO to deliver all Medicare hospital, physician, and nursing services while financing the additional in-home, community-based, long-term care services. Also included are such benefits as hearing aids, eye glasses, and prescription drugs.

The report states that the Social HMO project is continuing to meet two of its initial and ongoing challenges: financing and recruitment. Unlike many demonstrations, the Social HMO is paid for out of current premiums and service dollars rather than through research funds from HCFA. Despite this limitation, all sites are operating at the break-even point.

The project is currently focusing on these questions:

- Is it saving Medicaid funds by expanding long-term care benefits and integrated services? If so, how?
- Can it develop a new generation of Social HMOs that refine current approaches and extend the model to new populations?
- Can it determine who is really benefiting from the expanded long-term care services and case management efficiencies, and how this is being done?

The program currently rests at that point, with those and

other questions remaining to be answered, but its experience to date suggests that the eventual verdict will be favorable for at least some kind of Social HMO under the Medicare umbrella. I learned that much in May 1991, when I interviewed Lucy Nonnenkamp, director of the project at Kaiser in Portland.

She said that Congress is well enough impressed that it has extended the demonstration through the end of 1995, and has authorized its expansion to four additional sites. The site selection process is now being formalized.

Speaking for Kaiser Permanente, Lucy said her organization feels the Social HMO program has been fairly successful. It has kept many members out of nursing homes without going beyond its service targets or available funds. The community services have worked well through the end of 1990, but there is some reservation concerning the current year, as monthly premiums for the social HMO coverage have been increased from $75 to $125. Some members have dropped out for that reason, but membership of 5,400 is down only a bit from 6,100 at last year's end.

There are some restrictions on membership, such as a prohibition on residence in a nursing home, residential care facility, or foster care home at the time of enrollment, having end-stage renal disease requiring kidney dialysis, or being in hospice care. The other three sites also screen out all but 4 percent of applicants who are bed-bound or need assistance with activities of daily living.

Community care is an "everybody wins deal," Lucy said. "Not only does it meet a need, but it keeps people in their homes and lowers costs."

She added that Kaiser staff and enrollees are loyal to the organization and some have shown an interest in volunteering their services for certain community functions. The program has resource coordinators who go into the homes of frail members, and follow up at three-month intervals. If the members are receiving services, they get a call every month.

Many of the issues involved in the Social HMO experiment have not been addressed in this short study, because my purpose has been to describe the model and allow the reader to project how it interfaces with his or her own situation and community facilities. Some of these issues, which might prove to be controlling if extended to larger populations, will include:

- The problem of marketing the program to gain a large enough membership to make it workable in a given service area.
- Planning and providing for a minimum level of services, which must be expanded into areas in which traditional health service organizations may have little or no expertise.
- Developing criteria for quality controls, for reporting results for each level of service, and for extending or contracting the service portfolio to reflect actual demand in a given area.

It will be interesting to see what the future brings. The pioneers who have developed the Social HMO to this point have displayed a high level of perception, ingenuity and perseverance in putting the program together, and I suspect it will survive in some form or another for many years, perhaps as the model serving the elderly population best.

I persist in thinking, however, that there will remain many individuals and many communities that will not be served through a program designed for fairly large populations, and I shall continue my efforts to stimulate interest in helping those lonely, depressed, poor and sick elderly people through individual service and small local organizations. How might this be done? The next part, dealing with the prototype I call the "New Medicine Man," may provide part of the answer.

# Part II:
# The New Medicine Man

_The problems of older people are not just physical, but also mental and spiritual. Who is helping them to deal with these problems?_

Part II:
The New Medicine Man

# 13. Bridging the Gap

Where do the elderly turn for help when they develop the chronic ailments that plague so many when they pass the age of sixty, sixty-five, or seventy?

With few exceptions, they turn to their doctors. Granted, these ailments are most likely to appear initially as physical symptoms—high blood pressure, emphysema, gastric upsets, and so on. So it's logical to go to your doctor, right? And if he can't help you, who can? It seems logical—but might that logic be flawed?

This is what Marv Rosenberg, director for the Senior Peer Counselor Program for Group Health Cooperative of Puget Sound in Seattle, has to say:

"One of the things that concerns me most about current models of health care for the elderly is the dominant role those systems play outside the arena of physical health management. At an earlier time in history, one's ethnic or religious community and extended family provided the older person with emotional and home supports such as friendly visiting, safety checks, grocery shopping, home and yard maintenance, transportation, and so on. These days, the physician, social worker, physical or occupational therapist often finds himself or herself in the role of friend, confidant, and provider and coordinator of these services, thus spending valuable time on issues not related to physical health. The principle that drives the Senior Peer Counseling Program encourages the establishment of more appropriate supports for elders—outside the medical system— such as senior centers and neighbors that can take on some of the roles the extended family once provided.

"These elders may have lost their homes, many friends, perhaps their life partners, while their family members have scattered across the country. This leaves the older person increasingly isolated socially, but often well connected to the medical community where they get both social contact and health maintenance."

The way in which Group Health Cooperative is responding to this problem will be considered as one model program near the end of this section. But let us examine the shape of this problem further.

An important consequence of the absolute need of these elderly patients for some kind of social support is evident from a recent study of hospital readmissions I have reviewed. This study was done by a committee formed by a health maintenance organization (HMO) to determine what factors and costs are involved when patients are rehospitalized within a short time after being discharged. Are these readmissions necessary, and if so, why?

The study, covering a period of four months in late 1983 and early 1984, revealed that 100 readmissions occurred during that period. Of these, 30 had been planned at the time of discharge, so were not significant. Of the remaining 70 cases, 10 were patients who were readmitted *more than once* during a two-week period. Altogether, 51 patients were included in the review. Charts were available for 46 of those patients. Without going into detail as to the various diagnoses and causes for readmission, two things were especially striking about the study.

The first was the cost. The survey estimated that the total reimbursement for 50 cases could have been $222,267, based on the DRG codes (diagnosis-related groups) then in use. That is an average of $4,445 per case, incurred for an *unplanned* readmission following initial discharge.

The second major impact of the study comes simply from

glancing through the individual case records. These are most revealing. Here are a few, more or less typical, although there is no true norm for the highly individual situations:

• **CASE NO. 2:** Seventy-year-old woman with a long history of atherosclerosis, diabetes mellitus, obesity, status post CABG. Admitted with congestive cardiomyopathy and urinary tract infection. Past history of two carotid endarterectomies and left femoral-popliteal bypass surgery. Had CPR in past for episodes of ventricular fibrillation. Numerous notes in the chart referring to difficulty coping at home with medication and maintenance functions.

Admission history:
14 admissions since 1972
8 admissions in past 7 months
68 hospital days in past 7 months

• **CASE NO. 6:** Sixty-two-year-old woman admitted with recurrent vomiting for two weeks. History of left radical mastectomy in 1979 with subsequent recurrence and pleural effusion in December 1983. Two previous admissions since recurrence for control of nausea and vomiting. No consultation from hospice despite difficulties in coping with dying.

Admission history:
4 admissions since 1981
3 admissions in past 3 months
14 hospital days in past 3 months

• **CASE NO. 13:** Seventy-six-year-old woman with a subendocardial myocardial infarction, pulmonary edema, and atrial fibrillation on admission. History of multiple admissions for myocardial infarctions, congestive cardiomyopathy, pulmonary edema and cardiac arrhythmias. Patient lives alone, is anxious, and has a long history of dietary and medical non-compliance.

Reading through these dreary accounts, we frequently encounter such phrases as "family unable to cope with consequences," "history of severe financial difficulty," "lives with blind housekeeper—has anxiety over living situation and has difficulty coping with medication," "brought in because wife could not cope with consequences of these problems—patient bitter and depressed." So it's no wonder that, with no alternative social support program, these patients return to their doctors' offices and then their hospitals, again and again, because the pain of trying to cope with their devastated lives has become insupportable.

These two examples—the informed opinion of Marv Rosenberg and the revealing study of hospital readmissions—confirm this perception: People with physical impairments are channeled, often under some degree of duress, into the medical care system; while the same doctors, lacking training and skills in dealing with ailments that are wholly emotional, psychological, or spiritual, will turn patients with these non-physical complaints into counseling or religious channels. But with a few outstanding exceptions, which will be explored later in this section, there is no person or agency to bridge this gap—that is, to pull the physical and mental/spiritual treatment and healing modalities into one coordinated effort.

An individual patient who is not wholly satisfied with the degree of healing or recovery afforded by either system has the option of following a second track into the other system. But this can be very expensive, time-consuming, and counterproductive. We find these patients going to their own doctors and specialists for treatment of their tangible ills, while seeking help separately from an entirely different set of healers or counselors for intangible ills, although there may be only one set of causative factors for them all.

The patient may wind up many years later confused, considerably poorer, and not much better off in any respect. The common denominator is that the root causes of their problems, both physical and non-physical, may remain as potent as in the beginning, if not indeed more potent. The patients who do make it through the thicket of treatment, bills, late-night alarms, and prostrating panic attacks will usually have done it on their own. These are the fortunate few who educate themselves by sorting out the valid treatments from all those encountered, finally coming up with congenial and healthful regimens.

I think you have gathered, by this time, that appropriate health care for the elderly, more than for any other age group, involves attention to the whole person, body, mind, and spirit. The rationale and methods for such care are discussed in Parts III and IV. But first, we must look at existing systems and their practitioners to understand why and how they must be changed to make this possible.

Almost everyone gives lip service to the concept of holism (or wholism)—that is, comprehensive treatment of the patient's body-mind-spirit as a unit—but few are truly practicing it, and of these few, there are virtually none who are professionally educated and qualified to assess their patients' needs and to refer them to appropriate resources for treatment.

Of the medical doctors, the general practitioners and internists are the ones who are ostensibly trained in the broad symptomology of their patients' physical selves. Such training includes some backgrounding in psychology and mental illness —the brain and emotions playing prominent roles in many kinds of illness—but aside from this, these "family doctors" get a large share of their expertise in dealing with the intangible causes of illness simply from observation and experience.

When a patient passes beyond the care of his personal physician, he is usually referred to a specialist whose knowledge and skill are the most likely to be successful in dealing with the presenting symptoms. Sometimes the referral produces an optimal result, and the patient's symptoms are successfully abated. Sometimes two or more specialists get into the act before there is a conclusive result, but not infrequently there never is a true resolution regardless of the number of specialists consulted.

The psychiatrist is a medical doctor who deals with diseases of the mind, or the mind-brain. Like other doctors, his method of operation is to diagnose and treat the patient. This routine is often successful, but often it is not. Even when it succeeds, it is likely to be a long and expensive process, sometimes involving weekly sessions for two or three years at a cost of $75 per session or more.

The psychologist is a professional person, usually a doctor of philosophy (Ph.D.) trained to deal with mental and emotional problems that may or may not involve any physically debilitating symptoms. The psychologist may succeed through detailed interviews and counseling where no specific therapy or treatment is involved. The psychologist is usually not certified to prescribe drugs, but if he has clinical training he may recommend a drug to a referring physician.

These four types of professionals are the first line of health care for the average American with physical or mental dysfunctions, especially in view of the fact that medical insurance does not cover many diagnoses and treatments by practitioners outside this system. Why does this system of treatment result in such heavy use of prescription medications, and why are hospitals in the forefront of most health insurance programs when a very small proportion of illnesses actually require hospitalization?

I have been researching this problem for more than two years and have concluded that the answer lies in the way doctors are trained and the way elderly patients are compensated by Medicare for their treatments by doctors and hospitals. The treatment may be appropriate for purely physical ailments, but when mental and emotional ailments are included, as they often are, the doctors can do the only thing their education teaches them to do—write a prescription. They do on occasion make referrals to psychiatrists or psychologists, but this often takes the case beyond the doctor's control. And patients are prone to resist referrals if they feel they are being treated as "head cases," which has derogatory implications for most people.

The medical doctor is under the gun. Whatever his reasons for going into medicine in the first place—often altruistic, a genuine desire to help his fellow man—he learns from the beginning of his schooling that to succeed, he must go along with the unwritten, as well as the written, standards of his profession. These may include office location, equipment, staffing, hours and procedures; routines such as examinations, referrals, testing, charts and reports, supervision of hospitalizations and after-treatment, and the doctor's own continuing education;

participation in professional activities such as peer review, county, state, and national medical societies, legislative activities, civic enterprises, and so on. To be effective, both as a professional man and as a citizen, he must enjoy a certain income level and the cachet of a strong medical reputation. This is a tall order for any human to achieve.

One of the first things the doctor discovers is that he can't see enough patients to be a material success unless he cuts the minutes-per-patient call to a minimum, and charges at the high end of the scale permitted by society and the insurance companies. We're speaking directly of the family physician, or GP, although the same equation applies to most specialists. The latter, however, have a smaller patient base; they make up for this by allowing more time per patient, in most cases, and charging more dollars per call. At a time when my own family physician was charging $28 for a fifteen-minute office visit, I was referred to a skin specialist who charged $220 for a twenty-minute treatment. It's true I might have had more time for the same money, if I had needed it. The specialist, of course, charges because of his longer years of training, his specialized equipment—some of it very expensive—and his years of observation of a very narrow band of disorders.

I'll tell you a true story. My doctor had just bought himself a nice $28,000 Cadillac, for which I congratulated him. My dentist had told me about his jumping horses, which were not only expensive to maintain but which also led to his injuring his back and missing a few days of work. When I went to see the skin specialist mentioned above, I mischievously asked him if he owned a power boat.

"Oh, yes," he answered proudly, "and I also own a half interest in a place down at the beach."

I was glad to learn that I was one of that valiant band of patients who were keeping those three medical people in the toys they deserved.

The upshot of this time/dollar relationship, in the case of the general practitioners, is that few GPs have a true opportunity to deal with more than the presenting symptoms when a patient comes to them. Psychological factors are largely ignored. The history of the patient's family relationships, of job pressures, of extracurricular activities or after-hours capers, may find their way into a patient chart at the first interview, but are infrequently reviewed and pretty much forgotten upon the second and later calls.

I've had the experience of going to my doctor for a checkup, having him look quickly at my chart when he comes into the examining room, and say something like, "Let's see, now—the last time you were here we treated a hangnail. How is that coming?" The chances are that I had completely forgotten I ever had a hangnail. There may have been a dozen other blips and squiggles in my health story since then, but the doctor knows nothing about them. He never calls to ask how I am doing. His nurse never tells me to come in for a physical exam or a shot. I may have had several near-emergencies since the doctor last saw me, but if they aren't on my chart, they never happened, so far as he is concerned.

The doctor's whole training is directed at diagnosing and treating the patient's illness. Very little attention is paid to how the patient should manage or change his lifestyle, much less his habits and thought patterns, if this is needed for him to reach a higher level of health. The long speech with precise instructions about diet, rest, and exercise comes *after* the heart attack, not before.

Doctors themselves are the source of the most stinging indictments about the medical profession. You don't have to take my word for it. Here are some of the things they say:

❡ Doctors don't get enough training in pharmacology in medical school. The typical four-year training for a medical degree includes only one term of pharmacy and medication. After entering practice, most of what a doctor learns about pills comes from the detail men who represent the major drug companies. They call on him and give him brochures and samples of the medicines they are pressing him to prescribe.

❡ Doctors often give these free samples to patients having symptoms described in the brochures, hopeful that the pills will have the desired effects and that they (the doctors) can learn something about how the medicine works. Very often, the doctor is not adequately informed about how the medicine may affect older patients, with patients having other symptoms for which the pills are contraindicated (that is, recommended *against*), or with patients taking other medications that might have harmful interactions with the drug in question.

❡ Doctors are taught to end a typical interview by writing a prescription. The patient has come to expect it, and the doctor doesn't disappoint him. Very often, the drug chosen is simply a "best guess" on the part of the doctor—it may work to some degree, or it may cause discomfort or other unacceptable symptoms, or it may not work at all.

I've had the experience of reading about a new drug in a major magazine, mentioning it to my doctor, and having him give me a prescription for it without further investigation. I've also had another doctor prescribe two different drugs for my anxiety attacks (Triavil and Sinequan), neither of which worked in my case, only to wind up being sent to a clinical psychologist who suggested yet a third drug, Haldol. (This worked somewhat better, but made me very restless. I had to titrate it down to a tiny dosage, on my own initiative, before I could tolerate it.)

❡ Doctors don't have time to do all the studying and attend all the seminars they should to keep up with developments in their fields, which in the case of GPs, includes almost everything. They have been taught in medical school not to admit they don't know about a particular illness. Those who don't bluff outright may temporize, or make a diagnosis of "disease of the month," while they try one pill after another, or gossip around with other doctors and try to hit upon something that will keep the patient functioning. Nothing makes a doctor more cheerful than seeing an illness he can diagnose quickly and accurately, treat or prescribe for immediately, and have the patient's symptoms respond appropriately and disappear. Nothing upsets a doctor more than having a patient with an illness he can't recognize or diagnose, which his doctor friends can't help him with, and which keeps the patient showing up at the office or phoning several times a week.

You would think a doctor would be happy to see a patient like this take a hike and move his business to another doctor. Not so. The patient may be a pain in the neck, but the doctor likes to keep his business on the books, and the regular office calls may be money in the bank if they are covered by insurance or a solvent checking account. If a doctor loses very many patients, his reputation begins to suffer, not only among other patients but among other doctors as well.

There is a very substantial problem of impairment of doctors by the same stresses that bother so many of their patients. And the doctors, in too many cases, deal with these problems the same way the patients do—by denying their existence (to do otherwise would be to destroy the perception of their infallibility), to prescribe for themselves the same kinds of pills they prescribe for their patients, or to go the way of alcohol and street drugs. The "impaired doctor" syndrome is a major concern of the Oregon Board of Medical Examiners, which sponsors frequent seminars and courses aimed at airing and dealing with the problem.

(There are few solid statistics, but the figure of ten percent of doctors "impaired" to some degree is commonly accepted among those discussing the subject.)

As if all the foregoing strictures were not enough, the doctors of the land are limited by organizational structures and legal empowerments that afford them a large degree of professional protection while making innovation, departures from accepted practice, and movement between disciplines extremely difficult, or, in some cases, impossible. The system of medical education, licensing and board certification, internships and residencies in established hospitals, peer review, and related processes is one part of the picture. A second is the profession's own pyramid of county and state medical societies, topped by the American Medical Association, which have a tendency to keep doctors on a career track that might be threatened by any perceived heresy or just sheer contentiousness. And a third is the pattern of state legal requirements that change slowly, and that may act as a bar or damper to any doctor whose practice evolves too far from the accepted, even if outdated, norms.

Add to these comments another—that those doctors who become heavily involved in organizational duties and such paraprofessional activities as writing or TV appearances eventually drift into a bureaucratic or promotional mode, often bearing little relation to their purely medical competence. It is true that the preponderance of other doctors may look with some disdain at these medical politicos and lapel-mike wearers, but the latter are the ones the public hears and sees and who, by default, are usually accepted as the spokespersons for their entire professions.

At this point, I must offer a balancing opinion, which I hold just as strongly as those already expressed. This is that I like and admire medical doctors as a group very much. They are dedicated, they are sincere and professional, they work long, hard hours, they are serious in wanting to keep up-to-date in technical matters, and they are meticulous and caring in doing the best for their patients within the limitations of the system, which we have already explored. They are, for the most part, well qualified to provide the kind of treatment for which they are educated, and which their patients have come to expect. They are also, for the most part, businesslike and honest. There is little room in the profession for the lazy and unscrupulous, who are often tagged as such by their fellow doctors early in their careers. That being said, my earlier and following statements will stand as they are, unadorned.

# 14. Where Is Healing for the Spirit?

Well, if the medical profession, which includes psychiatrists, is untrained, inexperienced, and disinclined to become involved in the spiritual health of their patients, are the men and women of religion better prepared to deal with the physical health of their flocks (to put the matter of integrated health care into full perspective)? Or even to deal with their patients' spiritual ills?

The picture is far less clear in this area than in the medical/physical relationship. To be sure, there are some religious groups, such as the Christian Scientists, who see themselves as authorities for the total health needs of their flocks, but there is little acceptance for their views outside their own denominations.

To look beyond these rather specialized bodies, we naturally think of the various other churches and denominations as being in the front line of spiritual ministry. The poor ministers and priests are burdened at the outset with an insupportable cargo. If they head a congregation, they are expected to wear at least seven hats, and to be proficient in each responsibility, to wit:

First, as preachers. They must prepare and deliver a scholarly, well-researched, and eloquent sermon at least once a week, sometimes more often.

Second, as administrators and office managers. They must

head up the church office with all its responsibility for money handling, personnel supervision, duplicating, mailing, and so on.

Third, as fund-raisers and financiers. They must lead the planning and inspire the lay teams that raise the money for yearly operations as well as for long-term construction and equipment needs. The importance of this element of church life is apparent from the frequency with which ministers with a talent for fund-raising are hired to lead congregations that are at the point of raising funds for a new church building.

Fourth, as educators. They must not only be able to teach ethics and religion to adults and youth alike, but must see that the church's educational programs are properly staffed and carried out.

Fifth, as counselors. In this function, they come closest to serving as spiritual healers. But the nitty-gritty of the job means that they are often just picking up the pieces after the kid goes to jail, after the husband blows his brains out, or after the wife goes to Mexico with her old boyfriend. Consistent long-range counseling and soul-mending are virtually impossible for all but a select few obvious cases, usually those who come to the minister as a last resort.

Sixth, as organization leaders. They must oversee and support the myriad groups in a modern church—men's, women's, and youth—who carry out most of the congregation's social, developmental, and missionary functions.

Seventh, as visitors and church spokesmen. They must, after all, be ministers, visiting the ill, preaching at funerals, conducting baptisms and marriages, and serving as the representative of the church at all kinds of functions, however tenuous the relationship to their jobs.

Good heavens! How can one man or woman do all those things, and still find time for spiritual healing? The short answer is that they can't do it. Besides lacking the time, they do not have the skill or training, much less a perceived directive to perform this specific task. And for all their magnificent preaching, there are some in their flocks who misinterpret their words, like the boy who responded to a question about what he had learned from a parable by saying, "I want to be one of the multitude that loafs and fishes!"

This brings us to a delicate but obtrusive point. People trained as ministers may be very good at all the routine aspects of their jobs, but may be complete failures at the most important, which is being role models and guidance counselors in spiritual, moral, and ethical matters.

In my youth, my own family was served by five different ministers in five congregations. Of these, three "went bad." Two got themselves mired in financial difficulties, in both cases using church funds for unauthorized personal needs, the third leaving town in the company of a woman who was not his wife.

These experiences soured my father on the organized church, especially as *his* father had been a doctor of divinity and pastor of a large church in Philadelphia. It is difficult to say such experiences are atypical when they reflect a lifetime of affiliation with a particular denomination.

The point is an important one. As in the case of "impaired physicians," there are also "impaired preachers," and the recent cases of Jim and Tammy Bakker and Jimmy Swaggart are cases in point. There is no cachet in organized religion in America today for persons trained to deal full-time with the spiritual health of their public, as part of an integrated approach to total health—nor, perhaps, should there be. I shall discuss these mechanics later.

I am not taking account at this point of those who are "healers" first and ministers second. This would involve a discussion of the role of faith in healing and is beyond the scope of this paper. It is almost entirely outside the reach of traditional religious organizations.

The truth of these statements is seen readily in the experiences of ordinary church members who are ill and in need of help from whatever source—their doctors, various counselors and therapists, or their own ministers. Two or three times I have been visited by ministers while I was hospitalized. As I recall, these visits came at random times, were unsolicited and unexpected, and were too brief to accomplish anything. I did not know these people; they simply picked my name and "religious preference" off the hospital admission form. After a little small talk, and cursory questions about my health, the visitor would bow his head and say, "Shall we have a little prayer?" There would follow a nice and truly little supplication, having almost no bearing on my own situation, and the visitor would rise and take his leave, having achieved nothing but a pleasant, warm feeling in his own breast and, hopefully, in mine as well.

If you think I'm putting the worst face on the situation—that things aren't really as bad as all that—I'd like to balance the books by looking at some positive developments in the spiritual field.

The major religions do, indeed, play an important role in counseling in America. This bears not so much on health, but more on family life and personal crises, including ethical crimes that may have a spiritual connection. These services tend to be structural and organizational, but most ministers do as much as they can along these lines, considering competitive pressures for their time.

For example, some denominations, notably the Roman Catholic and Lutheran, are very active in providing counseling services. But they by no means dominate the counseling field, much less control it. Of some 315 listings in the Portland area Yellow Pages under "Counseling Services," only 24 appear to be church-connected. The Catholics and Lutherans each operate at several locations. There are other centers designated as "Christian," and one as a Latter Day Saints project. Most of the others among the 24 are individual churches, probably listed because of the commitment of a pastor or organization within those churches, or because the counseling service offers an outreach by the church to its community or potential clientele.

It is also clear from the names of counseling services that many do stress a spiritual approach, but from individualized viewpoints, such as the New Age, yoga, Inner Peace, etc.

There is also an ecumenical involvement in human reconstruction. For example, Oregon Ecumenical Ministries sponsors Project DARE (Drug and Alcohol Resources for the Elderly), which provides referrals to persons needing rehabilitation and support for substance abuse problems.

But ecumenism, the one movement that is body, mind, and soul into practical self-help for long-suffering humanity, is limited precisely because of its ecumenism: No participating preacher or lay person can say or practice anything that smacks of the sectarian, or doctrinal controversy, without facing the ire of the other supporting denominations. Proselyting is not just frowned upon; it is forbidden by the very nature of the ecumenical organization.

So how can ministers be better healers if they cannot inject their own beliefs, the fruits of their own education and training, if they are barred by the rules of engagement? At least in the ecumenical sphere, they can't—unless they speak solely from their own private pools of personal spiritual experience, and even for ministers that is sometimes a pretty small pool.

In defense of ministers, it will also be said that they do indeed provide a large measure of emotional and spiritual comfort to members of their flocks at times of crisis. And at their best, in such work as that of Dr. Norman Vincent Peale in his book, *The Power of Positive Thinking,* they have not only helped but changed lives by persuading people to place their lives in the hands of God. Without critiquing this process further, I point out only that it works best for those who have reached absolute bottom, and who are ready to trade their egos, their lifestyles, their habits and mindsets for peace of mind by letting God, through their consciences, make all their decisions for them. It is true this can and will work for anybody; but most individuals who have not fallen so far, or lost so much, will not readily or willingly take this radical step.

Beyond the medical doctor and the ordained minister, there is an almost unlimited spectrum of other disciplines and methodologies that offer to serve the person who is ailing in body, mind, or spirit. In general, they can be grouped under the heading of the holistic (or wholistic) movement, which has been with us for many years but seems to have been gathering momentum of late. Because it does not discriminate sharply between its attention to the three components of its human subjects—that is, body, mind, and spirit—I have chosen not to examine it in detail here, but in the following section, under the heading of healing modalities. I should say, however, that some of these modalities, especially those with Oriental origins, emphasize spiritual healing first, as a requisite for success in healing the mind and body. Yoga and Zen Buddhism are major examples, but spiritual healing is a component in virtually all the Eastern approaches.

Another way of looking at it is that the Eastern healers, and the traditional medicine men of nearly all primitive societies, have always linked the bodies, minds, and spirits of their subjects tightly together in their healing pursuits. Western medicine, as we have discussed, separates out the physical ailments (and some psychological ills) for treatment, leaving the health of the spirit to religious organizations or others. Are we right, and they wrong? There is no simple answer, but the philosophical basis of a possible solution will be considered in Parts III and IV of this book. But we must first complete our look at current ways of dealing with health matters.

# 15. The Paraprofessionals

It would not be proper to leave this consideration of society's healing apparatus without looking at yet a fourth area, in addition to organized medicine, organized religion, and the alternative approaches. This fourth area is quite diffuse, largely unrecognized as any kind of cognate group. They might be called the true paramedics—those without a formal, general education in medicine, yet people with great skills in healing owing to their long observation and experience, the depth of their reading, their relational talents, and a burning desire to help their long-suffering patients and clients.

These healers may have almost any kind of title to include large numbers of nurses, hospital and nursing home employees, social workers, physical therapists, massage technicians, athletic trainers, and others who simply grow into a healing role because of their insight into the needs of their charges, and their trial-and-error work in helping friends and associates through personal crises and toward better health.

They share this goal: To help and heal their clients, to free them from suffering, to get them well, to make them happy, and in a great many cases, to get involved in their lives as long-term friends and support givers.

People in this group are largely underpaid for this type of endeavor, at least on an hourly basis. But in the main, they do not crave material reward. Their compensation is in the health and happiness of their clients. They exchange Christmas cards, gifts, and messages of sympathy. They follow the comings and goings of whole families; they attend parties and celebrations together; they share information on health matters—new books and articles, new theories, new foods and medicines, and so on. They are forever photocopying something for a relative or friend who may need the type of information it contains.

They are generally innovative and open to experiment. They adhere to the sports dictum: Never change a winning game, always change a losing game. They know the value of placebos, whether these be actual pills or simply a different exercise regimen. They know the values of right thinking and clear consciences. They know what happens when people become fixated on negative goals, or fearful of taking a positive step in any direction. They are perceptive and attentive to the signals given out by their clients that may indicate spiritual distress as well as physical and mental symptoms. To some degree, they fulfill the role of the medicine man in primitive societies. Yet in the main, they lack the cachet of a medical degree, and usually lack the technical training to provide more than loving support and a degree of comfort and reassurance.

To be fair, there are some danger signals that one should be alert to. There's the former neighbor who may be making a living selling health food products or home remedies. There's the zealous friend whose "problems" have been cleared up by magnets or crystals, although these may have performed only as placebos. There's someone else who has heard of a doctor in Colorado who can heal just about anything by a special kind of acupuncture. And so on. Anyone who is in business full-time to serve and treat patients needs some kind of organizational certification to be accepted as genuine; and one must always view their claims with dispassionate reserve until they have been given a trial.

The point is, I think, that no one has a monopoly on truth. The wise client or patient will observe an operating rule I learned in a college logic class: When the experts agree on something, the wise person is loath to hold an opposing opinion; when the experts disagree, the wise person withholds final judgment. In applying this to modern medical problems, as reported in the media, most of us (if we are indeed wise) are probably withholding judgment on a wide range of matters, because there seems to be scant agreement among the experts on anything.

Where does this leave elderly patients, who may have learned most of what they know about health when they were still living at home with their parents? Exactly as I described them in Part I—too many of them lonely, ill, confused, and lacking the skill and energy to help themselves. This is the point at which we should be looking to new models, and new theories, to reach a solution.

Enter the New Medicine Man!

# 16. Who Is the New Medicine Man?

So we come down to the question: Who is the New Medicine Man? What's new? Is he a doctor? Is he, perhaps more to the point, a witch doctor? Is he a healer? Is he part of the medical establishment, or the religious establishment, or the hospital or HMO establishment—or *any* establishment? Does he go to a New Medicine Man college and earn a New Medicine Man license? Is this a full-time job? Does he get paid—and if so, how? With whom, if anybody, does he compete?

I shall not attempt to answer these questions directly, or in order, but instead shall give my own opinions, definitions, and recommendations as though I were describing a new organism. In the course of doing so, I hope the reader will understand how it all fits into the present scheme of things. I think this can happen without creating major disruptions, or the need to change immediately anything that is already being done. Instead, if it works as I know it can, it should catalyze systems already in place to do a lot of better work for less money, to make things easier for professionals and support systems who are heavily stressed, and to provide answers to many of the most pressing questions of the elderly needy, hungry, and ill without taking anything away from anybody else.

The New Medicine Man, of course, is gender-neutral. I use

the male form partly for convenience, simply to represent a prototype, and partly to avoid the necessity of using he-or-she, him-or-her, or his-or-hers every time I need a pronoun.

But beyond that, the New Medicine Man represents more than the knowledge or talent of a single individual. He really acts as a gateway to all the technical knowledge and skill, all the awareness and support, all the positive reinforcement and love that a patient needs to reach a stable, self-controlled condition of true health.

The New Medicine Man will not be a person who necessarily takes a prescribed course of study in a professional school, receives a certificate of proficiency, and spends a certain period of time in institutional practice, internship, or apprenticeship. He may or may not have had medical training per se, but he will be knowledgeable about modern medical practice and problems, and the ways in which this practice impinges on the lives of older patients. He will have studied, read widely and had practical experience in such fields as philosophy and ethics, counseling and rehabilitation, alternative therapies and psychology, as well as the well-known schools of politics, business, and hard knocks. He will most probably be retired. His motivation will rise from his observation of the imperative needs of elderly relatives, friends, and neighbors who are victims of the present-day structure of our medical and care systems, with the skewed decisions enforced by the related payment schedules, especially Medicare. His working life may have been spent in medicine, counseling, social work, operating nursing homes, or running agencies involved with human services. He probably will not have begun with the overt purpose of being a New Medicine Man at all.

At some point shortly before or after retirement, he will become aware of the relatedness of physical, mental, and spiritual problems as they affect his elderly friends, perhaps including his spouse, his living parents, his brothers and sisters, and other near relatives. If he has been involved directly with services to the elderly, he will have seen the shortcomings of the system that funnels them either into medical channels, on the one hand, or the "soft" disciplines of psychology and religion, on the other. He will see the need for bridging this gap, and will be sharply aware that he himself has many of the skills needed to bring resources and patients together, and to blend the services of the medical and support communities. This means that, ideally, he should combine these attributes:

1. He should be widely informed in the disciplines that deal with the three components of human health: body, mind, and spirit.
2. He must be a person of maturity and experience, sensitivity and humility, unquestioned integrity and perpetual optimism, and good humor.
3. He must be alert to the moods and feelings of his clients, and be a good "reader" of their reactions to his questions and to their own perceptions.
4. He must be a communicator par excellence, with access to a network of professionals and agencies in the health field, able to elicit information and to gain cooperation.
5. He must have a burning desire not merely to help others, but to complete his own spiritual growth by willingly letting go of his own ego demands, his own need for recognition and material reward, and to replace them by the knowledge that he is born again every day into new opportunity for learning and service.

I hope I haven't scared too many readers away by this idealized portrait. I've painted that picture as a goal that might be held in view by anyone choosing to travel this path, knowing that the start will be from a much more modest platform. And to prove that this is not an impossible goal, I offer two models, involving senior peer counselors, that are up and running and entirely successful.

The first of these is the Stephen Series, founded in 1975 by a St. Louis pastor with a background in psychology. It is named for St. Stephen, a follower of Christ known for his interest in serving the poor, widows, and orphans. Despite its recent inception, the ministry is already functioning in more than 3,000 parishes and congregations throughout the United States.

The ministry requires participating caregivers to adhere to rigorous guidelines embodied in a massive policy manual. The lay caregivers are trained to follow these principles in dealing with older citizens who are referred to them:

1. Do not give advice.
2. Do not suggest cures.
3. Do not recommend any particular service or treatment.

The Stephen ministers in any given congregation are set up under a coordinator, who works with a few small teams, each with a leader, and each with about six members who work one-on-one with a care receiver.

The primary tool of the workers is careful listening, buttressed by the ability to recognize the importance of feelings. The leaders also train their Stephen ministers in assertiveness, and give the church's pastors feedback that will be of use in their pastoral work. This feedback, however, never violates the confidentiality of the relationship.

The Stephen ministers spend at least one hour each week with their assigned care receivers. The purpose of this is to keep the work from becoming too onerous or overwhelming, or so extensive that care receivers become dependent. Another aim is to keep the Stephen ministers from identifying so closely with their care receivers that they draw personal power from the relationship.

The Stephen ministers do not provide services themselves, but make referrals to health providers or other agencies, such as Meals on Wheels, public transportation companies, or congenial support groups.

Work on any given care relationship can run from three months to a year, but in the absence of a resolution of the situation at the end of that time, the care receivers are referred to some kind of continuing care agency.

Other principles are aimed at getting the care receivers to take initiatives to help themselves; to assign ministers to care receivers of the same gender; to treat all work in absolute confidence; and to locate respite resources for other caregivers, such as the spouses of the care receivers.

There is no set number of individual ministers for one congregation, but two dozen or more would not be uncommon. In larger cities where there are several churches operating a program, there is usually an informal network whose leaders meet every three months or so to share information and ideas. Stephen ministers are occasionally traded between churches to ensure better matches between ministers and care receivers.

Stephen ministers pay their own expenses, although their churches may cover their initial training and national program fees. Groups in some cities publish newsletters to help churches stay up to date and follow common policies. Prospective care receivers are referred to the churches by many sources, and need not be members of a given church.

The Stephen Series obviously does not conform in all respects to the principles I outlined earlier, but it does meet the all-important Number One: providing a trained peer caregiver who goes into the home of an elderly person in need of support, listens to the stories and complaints of that person, then tries to locate the resources to deal with them. If this organization follows through on its policies and goals, it cannot fail to achieve a substantial measure of success.

In operation, the ministry achieves nearly as many benefits for its participants as for its care receivers. The extensive and rigorous training, followed by the months of rewarding service, give continuing satisfaction to both parties. I checked with a nearby church that has such a program, and learned that the ranks of ministers are not only well filled, but those volunteering include many of the "pillars of the church." A friend who made name tags for them told me he was surprised at the caliber of these people. He said they were also carefully screened, so there is little possibility that the program will be abused.

The second model of a successful senior peer counselor program we'll look at is that of the Group Health Cooperative of Puget Sound, operated in the Seattle area under the directorship of Marv Rosenberg, who was quoted earlier. He has a master's degree in social work, and has been working in the field of senior care for the past fifteen years. This program has filled many of the roles I prescribed as the functions of a "New Medicine Man," although it is somewhat more limited, and of course confined to the organizational umbrella of the Group Health Cooperative.

Unlike other models in which another piece of medical support is added, the Group Health plan enters a client's care program in a transient or temporary mode, usually four to six months. The goal of the senior peer counselor is not to become a lifelong friend of the elderly client, but to help identify more appropriate sources of social support rather than continuing to go through the medical community.

If the clients have moved away from their former neighborhoods, this program helps to get them linked back to their families as well as their new neighborhoods. This encourages the community to begin to support the older people in the place of their doctors. It's the shop owner, the grocery store manager, the beautician, or someone else within the natural orbit of the client who may be enlisted to provide that missing personal link. Perhaps someone on the staff of the nearest senior center can take a hand and help line up support.

These contacts, arranged as early as possible following the client's arrival in his or her new community, can help people to mourn the death of a partner who had a chronic illness. This is especially important if the surviving client was a full-time caregiver who had already let go of existing supports in the old setting. See what has happened: The caregivers have lost their own personal contacts, as well as a sense of place and purpose, because their own skills as caregivers are no longer needed. There is also pride involved. They were not trained to be caregivers, but they learned, and did their best, and perhaps feel they have failed because the spouse died.

For clients who were business or professional people before they retired, they may no longer identify with their earlier persona. There has to be a readjustment. If that had not happened when the spouse became ill, the survivor may have become a "professional" caregiver, and when that job is lost through death of the spouse, it doubles the sense of failure.

The senior peer counselor tries to get into that situation before it develops. Many clients, including most of those with Alzheimer's disease and other degenerative ailments, are reluctant to listen to professionals who are younger than they, and who haven't had experience to match theirs. They may also fail to understand or really to "hear" what their doctors tell them.

The peer counselors are in the same age bracket as their clients. Some of them may also have lost a spouse to Alzheimer's. Such a person can tell his client, "Look, I see the signs of what's coming. I know what's likely to happen, and I think I can help you prepare for it." Having gained the respect and confidence of the client, the peer counselor can then suggest options. If there is a caregiver involved, one solution might be to get temporary help to provide the caregiver with respite. Or the client might be placed in a skilled nursing facility for a while.

The Group Health senior peer counselors are all volunteers. What the organization looks for are retired persons such as professionals, social workers, psychologists, nurses, senior center administrators, personnel directors, and "people people" such as recreation leaders. People like this understand human behavior and needs.

Rosenberg cited an example of a peer counselor who had retired after many years working as a seamstress in a major department store. She said her work had prepared her to become a peer counselor, because she developed the skill of making people comfortable and at ease while working with them "up close and personal."

Senior peer counselors receive thirty hours of training provided by Rosenberg and the Group Health staff. Training topics include communication skills, counseling techniques, dealing with loss and grief, crisis intervention, and an in-depth orientation concerning the two dominant mental health problems of the elderly: depression and anxiety. The volunteers meet twice a month to consult with Rosenberg and each other regarding their clients, and ways of presenting solutions to gain acceptance from their clients. After the initial training, volunteers receive on-going training and supervision after they start working with clients.

The only requirement of clients is that they be enrollees in the

Group Health plan, in addition to being at least fifty-five years of age. The counselors have the option of giving their phone numbers to their clients, to be used only in emergencies, but the clients can always call Rosenberg if their counselor is not available. The peer counselor is matched carefully with the client to make compatibility most likely. One of the first things Rosenberg did after receiving funding for the program was to establish an advisory board to shape it. The board was made up of older consumers, medical providers, and administrators. There were fifteen senior peer counselors at the time I talked to Rosenberg; the policy is to assign two or three clients to each.

There has been no significant problem in finding counselors. Rosenberg runs notices in *View* magazine, Group Health's own publication. He also sends fliers to senior centers, and runs articles in local newspapers and publications such as *Source Magazine*, an organ of the Seattle Council of Churches. Volunteers fill out applications; Rosenberg then interviews them by telephone, and if there is continued interest on both sides, a face-to-face interview is scheduled. They are asked to sign up for a minimum of six months' work after completing training; anything longer is a bonus, Rosenberg says, because by then they will have justified the time spent in training.

There are benefits to the senior peer counselors. They find the work exciting. They have become "street smart" from their own experiences, and they are willing to face problems involving death or other emergencies. They don't have to be members of Group Health, but nearly all of them are.

There's the inevitable administration for Rosenberg. Peer counselors must make written reports of their contacts with clients, which Rosenberg reviews to assure the volunteers are conducting themselves appropriately and the clients' needs are being addressed. In addition, there is the usual report writing, statistical compilations, and quality assurance work connected with running the program.

Peer counselors have certain limitations. Although many of them are retired professionals, they are not permitted to provide professional advice or services. As volunteers, they cannot make medical or psychiatric assessments or determine treatment plans. They must refer their clients back to the health care system for this. However, peer volunteers can bring valuable information back to Rosenberg and the clients' health care team regarding the clients' functioning. The peer volunteer can also provide emotional support, act as a bridge to link the client with the appropriate resources, and work with the client to develop methods of tackling problems and recognizing options.

Group Health members can now ask that a peer counselor be assigned to them; in the beginning, they came by professional referral only.

There has been enough experience to convince Rosenberg and other staff members that Group Health is saving not only money, but also the time of medical staff and other resource personnel who previously had to provide support.

If you will compare the operations of the Group Health model of senior peer counselor, you will see that it parallels very closely the qualifications I spelled out earlier in this part of defining the New Medicine Man. About the only difference is that the Group Health people operate under an organizational umbrella, while the prototype of the New Medicine Man will be a self-starter who manages his own program, seeks out his own clients, and makes his own rules and regulations. Because of an assumed similarity of backgrounds, however, my guess is that there would be few real differences in terms of client relations and benefits. I'd just like to see a lot more of both on the American scene!

After I had gathered all my material for this part of the book, and written most of it, I had an idea that would enable the concept of the New Medicine Man to be put into operation immediately, without a lot of planning and preparation.

Nearly every hospital in the country has some kind of volunteer organization, which does such things as deliver patient mail, distribute magazines and books and other comfort items, push wheelchairs, help with administration, and so on. Some of these volunteers are older people, whose physical strength may be limited but whose time and enthusiasm are not. A few of these volunteers could be picked for training as senior peer counselors to provide exactly the kind of support that the study of hospital readmissions, reported earlier, found to be lacking in the homes of many elderly patients following their release. The hospitals can identify these patients without great effort, and I think would be well rewarded by having a peer counselor check on them at home for three or four days after leaving the hospital. The counselors could spend enough time with each patient to hear all their problems and complaints, to uncover the fears and inhibitions and reticences, and to try to figure out what resources and further supports might be needed to enable the patients to stay at home without having to return to the hospital.

Then, in cases involving an obvious need for a change of life management, such as a move to an adult foster care home, the counselor would be in position to begin negotiations with the appropriate agency and to persuade the patient and/or the concerned relatives to acquiesce in sound decisions. Sources of funds would have to be identified as those of the patient, available insurance coverage, charitable programs, or public resources.

I think such a movement would also clarify the need to get some of these things done earlier in the game, before these painful crunches develop. Everyone—doctors, agencies, hospitals, and caregivers—should see the advantage of making earlier choices and developing other action plans before the hospitals found themselves with these old, sick, and, in many cases, dying patients on their hands. I can't go into greater detail without further research and consultation, but it's certainly worth thinking about.

# Part III:
# The Art of Healing

*¶  Only when you are fully healed
are you fully free.*

# 17. My Travels in Drugdom

Friday, May 13, 1960, did *not* start just like any other day. Just the reverse; it started like no other day in my life.

I woke up at 2:30 A.M. with my heartbeat out of control. My heart was flopping around in my chest like a flounder in the bottom of a rowboat. I was certain at first that I was having a heart attack, but I grew less certain as each minute passed. There was no pain, and there was no dimming of my senses, no lack of ability to get up and move around. But I suffered extreme nervousness, and finally, fear.

What I was having, I later learned, was a classic bout of atrial fibrillations. The atria are the two upper chambers of the heart, which receive blood from the veins and in turn force it into the ventricles. The latter, the two lower chambers, receive blood from the atria and pump it into the arteries, then throughout the body, supplying oxygen and nourishment to the cells.

Any continued lapse of function of the atria would, of course, decrease the efficiency of the heart because the atria and ventricles would be out of rhythm, and delivery of blood to the body would be affected. But occasional bouts of atrial fibrillation, if not long continued, are not especially damaging.

I didn't know any of this on that fine day in May, thirty years ago. I was alone on the first floor of our Cape Cod house in northeast Portland, Oregon, because my wife Erma had gone to Tacoma to be with our daughter for the birth of our first grandchild. Our two sons, Jim, seventeen, and David, thirteen, were asleep upstairs.

If then were now, I'd have gone to the telephone and dialed 911. I suppose I should have tried to reach my doctor, or called Portland Adventist Hospital, about two miles away. Instead, I waited. I was reluctant to wake the boys, who were not trained in CPR and probably would not have been able to do much anyway, as that kind of fibrillation is not susceptible to first aid measures. Jim would have had to drive me to the emergency room at the hospital, but I didn't feel a need for that.

I tried to compose myself, lying flat on my back and breathing as slowly and deeply as I could. I moved my limbs cautiously, then got up and walked around, thinking that perhaps this movement would pull my heart back to normal. No luck.

So I just lay there in bed and worried. About what could possibly be happening to me. About whether I'd have to get Erma to come back from Tacoma immediately. About how I was going to get all my work taken care of. About all my other family and community obligations. And about what my world would be like if I survived this thing. Would I be an invalid or a cripple? Would I live a few days, then die? I have to tell you, my thoughts were mostly selfish, and I had not yet begun to think about what would happen to my family, relatives, and friends if I were no longer around.

But as you have no doubt guessed, I didn't die, or I would not be writing these lines. At 9 A.M., my elder son drove me to my doctor's office. I was then driven to a nearby hospital, where bedrest, tranquilizers, and quiridine had me back on my feet in one day.

So what was my problem? How did I handle it, how did I finally overcome it, and how does it relate to this book?

To be brief, I was a classic victim of stress, and I was having a classic reaction. There was also a subplot: as my doctor told me later, most people can handle stress if it occurs mainly on the job, while they enjoy tranquility at home. Or they can handled stress at home, if their jobs are running smoothly. But if they are heavily stressed both at home and on the job, one of three things will happen. They'll have ulcers, high blood pressure, or a heart attack.

Without going into detail, I fell into the last category. I was working for a demanding boss who felt the best way to get the most out of his employees was to keep them buried with work. And on the home front, my daughter had married a young man of whom, to use the mildest possible term, my wife and I did not approve. When the new husband reenlisted in the army and headed for Germany without my daughter, we had her back on our hands for three more years, off and on. Daughter gave birth to her first-born, husband returned from Germany, daughter had another child, later attempted suicide, and divorce followed. Join the club!

I got through the first episode of fibrillations without serious complications or continuing medication. But after a second episode in the spring of 1963, I wound up on quinidine sulfate to prevent heart arrhythmias.

The stress continued, along with the tension, anxiety, and panic attacks. In October 1963 I consulted an industrial physician who gave me the Minnesota Multiphasic Personality Inventory (MMPI), decided I wasn't mentally unbalanced, and prescribed Stelazine, a major tranquilizer. I continued on that until the end of 1978. Meanwhile, in July 1964 I also began taking Valium to reduce my tension and to help me sleep better. That also continued until 1978.

But the course of true stress never runs smooth. I finally solved the work problem by taking a fairly stress-free job in 1970, and in 1976 I retired, after forty-one years in newspaper, advertising, and public relations work. I had also spent nearly thirty-four years in the army reserve, during the last sixteen of which my two weeks of active duty every summer was also my annual vacation. Our sons were graduated from college, had married, and started families. Their domestic problems were less stormy than my daughter's, but there were problems. I also discovered, as have many others, that there are stresses associated with retirement that few people foresee.

Despite all my medication, I had some rough times in late 1978 and early 1979, and in the summer of 1980 the whole thing came crashing down around me when my Dalmane (a replacement pill for Valium) apparently quit working, and I tried to withdraw, cold turkey, on my own. I suffered a full-blown breakdown, with heavy night sweats, hallucinations, tachy-cardia, disabling weakness, convulsions, insomnia, and two or three other symptoms.

After three months in bed, I switched to a new doctor. He was a stress specialist, and immediately put me on Tranxene, a drug in the same family as Valium and Dalmane. All are benzodi-azepines. They work by substituting a molecule of their own for one of the body's neurotransmitters, which bind to nerve recep-tors and prevent panic signals from getting through to the heart, muscles, and other organs.

I perceived at the time that my own natural stress-fighting mechanism had become functionally atrophied because the pills were doing all the work, and this was borne out when I stopped the Dalmane and had all that trouble. The Tranxene reversed it, and I felt better again. But black moods and depression re-turned. I sensed that all the old emotional "garbage" was still buried there in my subconscious.

Beginning in January 1981 my doctor turned me over to his stress management therapist, Karen Mahan. She knew what to do. Gently, with a combination of biofeedback and a psycholog-ical discipline called mentation, she helped me get rid of my hang-ups and regain my normal energy and optimism to a major degree.

I stayed on medication for another six years. But for nine months in 1987, with Karen's help and a new technique using a computer to monitor my breathing and heart rate, I was able to stop all the pills, taking the last half of a Digoxin tablet on October 27, 1987. All during those nine months, the old with-drawal symptoms would reappear, one by one, and would be sloughed off, like the layers of skin from an onion. Each time I decreased the dosage, I'd suffer through the symptoms until I stabilized, then went on to the next lower dosage. I came off Tranxene, Digoxin, and Quinaglute in that way, and I haven't had any of those pills since.

Among the things I realized during that long seven years of recovery was that my major foe, all along, had not been the stress itself, but fear—fear of having a heart attack. This was surely based on my original doctor's statement that, if I continued to be doubly stressed at work and at home, I would have high blood pressure, ulcers, or heart trouble. Because of the fibrillations, I had decided subconsciously that I was going to have a heart attack, and I had been waiting for one ever since.

Through counseling, I also realized other things: that I was a free person, and was not bound by any laws or rules that could inhibit my actions, communications, or thoughts; that I could do anything in my life I wanted to do, if I would just establish and hold onto a goal (but that I could never do *everything*); that I had no enemies, and no one was conspiring against me, unless I chose to make this happen; that there was nothing essentially wrong with my heart or body, and I could use them up to my capacity without worrying about damaging them.

Along the way, Karen taught me how to use biofeedback skills such as skin warming and control of breathing to attain relaxation. By that method I overcame an attack of vasomotor rhinitis, two or three bouts of arthritic pain and weakness, and several incipient sore throat/cold sequences that just never got started.

I hope you won't interpret this account of my experience as a statement of any superior knowledge or ability on my part, much less as an intention to convince you that I have the keys to health and long life, which I want you to buy from me. By no means. I do want you to understand that I am not writing solely on the basis of academic research, or of reading and conversations with others. I'm not shooting blanks. I've suffered the maladies of the times along with everybody else. As I write, I'm facing surgery to implant radioactive "bullets" of Iodine-125 in my prostate to shrink, and hopefully destroy, a malignant nodule there. I have full confidence in the doctors who are treating me, and I am thankful for the skills and technology that give me a good prognosis. But the solutions I found for many of my other ills have been appropriate for me if not for others. These experiences have been real; I've felt and seen the maladies come and go. I'm not saying anything I don't know from having been through it myself, or haven't validated with others. I have spoken to many groups about my dependence on drugs, including an appearance on a panel on drugs and the elderly at the 1991 conference of the National Council on Aging in Miami. I have yet to be challenged on anything I have said, and I think this is because I speak from the heart, and speak only of things I know to be true from my own experience. Information I have gathered by reading or interview is attributed to the sources indicated.

To get my own thinking from where I was at the end of 1987, when I completed withdrawal from pills, to where it is today, after two years of research into the strengths and weaknesses of modern medicine, we have to look at the actual course of this research. I began by studying the problem of overmedication and mismedication of the elderly, which had been at the root of my own problem; that is, the tendency to rely on pills to solve conditions of the mind and spirit that really couldn't be solved in that way. I soon saw that this state of affairs could be traced to the medical establishment, supported by conditioning of the public, which relied on the philosophy that the way to deal with human illness is to diagnose and treat it on a symptom-by-symptom basis, as one would repair an automobile. It followed that the only way to get back to a whole-person approach to true health would be to formulate new models for health care, especially for older people, whose illnesses tend to be chronic, and interwoven with psychological and emotional factors.

# 18. How Did We Get Here?

A few paragraphs on the nature of our present health predicament are needed to bring it into focus. Since the beginnings of modern medicine, which can be traced back to the Greek, Hippocrates, and beyond, treatment for illness followed a holistic model, one that regarded human beings as complex entities made up of body, mind, and spirit. In an earlier era, and in primitive societies today, the assistance of the gods was invoked to drive out evil and permit natural healing processes to work. Hippocrates and the other physicians of his time, however, held that illnesses are *not* caused by supernatural forces, but are natural phenomena that can be studied scientifically and influenced by therapeutic procedures and by wise management of one's life.

The Greek physicians of that era, as revealed in their writings, show in great detail how the well-being of individuals is influenced by environmental factors—the quality of air, water, and food, the topography of the land, and general living conditions. The understanding of environmental effects was seen as the essential basis of the physician's art. Thus health was considered to be a balance among environmental influences, ways of life, and the various components of human nature.

Hippocrates recognized the healing forces inherent in living organisms, forces he called "nature's healing power." The role of the physician was to assist these natural forces by creating the most favorable conditions for the functioning of the healing process.

The theories of Hippocrates and his contemporaries paralleled, in some ways, the medical doctrines and practices of the Chinese from their first efforts to formalize them and record them. But the Chinese were less interested in causative factors in illness than in relational factors—that is, the subject's position relative to other human beings, his community, and the natural setting in which he lived. Thus a person's health reflected the harmony in which he and his social and natural environment existed, and illness was disharmony at the individual and social levels.

In the Chinese view, according to Fritjof Capra, author of *The Turning Point,* the individual is responsible for the maintenance of his own health, and to a great extent, also for the restoration of health when the organism gets out of balance.

Without going into the subtle differences between Eastern and Western medicine, and the religious and superstitious elements that attended medical practice between the time of the Greeks and the late Middle Ages, it is enough to say that there were no real divergences in views toward medicine until the scientific upheavals of the sixteenth and seventeen centuries— roughly the period during which Galileo, Descartes, and Newton made their observations and propounded their theories. The net outcome of their discoveries, in terms of their effect on medicine, was the continuing attempt to reconcile medical practice with changing views of the universe, the world itself, and of human life and physiology. The so-called "Cartesian method" that influenced development of the "hard sciences" grew out of Descartes' belief that "all science is certain, evident knowledge. We reject all knowledge which is merely probable and judge that only those things should be believed which are perfectly known and about which there can be no doubt." The rigorous application of this scientific method led to a further dictum, which is known as reductionism. This is the belief that "all complex phenomena can be understood by reducing them to their constituent parts."

You can see what the literal application of these views would have done to the theory and practice of medicine, and indeed to all the other so-called "soft" sciences such as psychology, sociology, politics, and economics. It would have reduced them to mathematical formulae based on tables of statistical observations, and would have resulted in a number of absurdities along with the occasional valuable insights that occurred. To a considerable extent, this happened. It had an impact on medicine and the healing arts, resulting in a real if indistinct split between "mainstream medicine" and the alternative methods, which will be discussed later in this section. Medical doctors have always recognized the existence of psychological, emotional, and spiritual factors beyond the scope of their training, and the alternative practitioners have likewise recognized the priority of good physical examinations, diagnoses, and treatment. But attempts to pull them together into a true "holistic" mode have not been very successful to date.

By the time this century opened, the scientific revolution had built up such a head of steam that it had swept most other fields of study into its orbit. The major exception was the field of religion, or theology, which kept to its own traditions and literature, and was recognized by the academics only as a completely separate and totally mystic kingdom, inaccessible by any of the standard "scientific" means of verification and extrapolation. In this time period, we have seen many largely irrelevant attempts to certify religious "facts" by scientific methods, such as determining the origin of the Shroud of Turin, photographing reported appearances of the Virgin Mary, trying to ascertain whether the tears and blood appearing on crucifixes were real, and so on. The problem here is not whether these phenomena are real in scientific terms, but whether the findings can or should affect the beliefs of those who are influenced by them. (For myself, I'd just as soon that events that I hold to be mystical *not* be photographed or pinned to a board like a butterfly.)

Recently, many writers, including Capra, have referred to the Cartesian, or reductionist, approach to medicine as the biomedical model, or perhaps more graphically, the biomechanical model. The weaknesses of this approach are spelled out by Capra in these words:

The human body is regarded as a machine that can be analyzed in terms of its parts; disease is seen as the malfunctioning of biological mechanisms which are studied from the point of view of cellular and molecular biology; the doctor's role is to intervene, either physically or chemically, to correct the malfunctioning of a specific mechanism. Three centuries after Descartes, the science of medicine is still based, as George Engel writes, on "the notion of the body as a machine, of disease as the consequence of the breakdown of the machine, and of the doctor's task as repair of the machine."

By concentrating on smaller and smaller fragments of the body, modern medicine often loses sight of the patient as a human being, and by reducing health to mechanical functioning, it is no longer able to deal with the phenomenon of healing. This is perhaps the most serious shortcoming of the biomedical approach. Although every practicing physician knows that healing is an essential aspect of all medicine, the term "healer" is viewed with suspicion, and the concepts of health and healing are generally not discussed in medical schools.

I think most doctors would agree that this is an extreme and oversimplified view of the way modern medicine is practiced, but it does explain why they are reluctant to go beyond diagnoses and methods of treatment that have been validated by scientific means.

There were other by-products of the scientific model. One of these was the germ theory, which followed the discovery of disease-producing organisms by Louis Pasteur in the latter part of the nineteenth century. Then in the twentieth century came the discovery of Salvarsan, a cure for syphilis; the sulfa drugs for treatment of various infections; penicillin, a broad-spectrum derivative of a mold for many more types of infections; the Salk and Sabin vaccines for poliomyelitis; and finally, the mind- and mood-altering drugs, chemical controls for nervous disorders, and a host of other "magic bullet" treatments for many previously "incurable" diseases.

All of these developments reinforced the belief that illnesses were biomechanical and could be controlled or cured by specific, one-shot, tangible agents, if only those agents could be identified.

Concurrently, surgery likewise made great strides, abetted by continuing improvements in anesthetics and the proliferating diagnostic procedures such as X-rays, followed by the exploding technology of lab tests, blood manipulation, organ transplants, heart by-pass surgery, and so on. All this at tremendous cost in public and private dollars, justified on the theory that no cost is too great to save a human life, or indeed to improve the quality of the lives saved and prolonged.

This healing development has been abetted since World War II by new theories of public responsibility and social support for maintaining the health of individuals. The Hill-Burton Act of the mid-1940s provided matching funds for construction of hospitals nationwide; no self-respecting small town could stay in business without a well-equipped modern hospital, it seemed. Public health services were extended to populations that had previously received little or no care at all. Private health insurance, often subsidized or fully provided by employers, became a prized benefit of employment. And finally, in the mid-1960s the Great Society of the federal administration produced Medicare and Medicaid, extending health coverage to vast new numbers of the elderly and the indigent.

These developments, on top of the expensive new technology, brought about an exponential increase in the cost of health care, described in Chapter 2. All these considerations raise perplexing issues of public policy that are reflected in decisions that have to be made by individuals as well as by politicians, public employees, and businessmen. The key issues, of course, are how much health care is too much, and where a line should be drawn as to what our society can afford. The question as to whether individual citizens are entitled to all the health care they wish to pay for is relevant, asking whether the well-off should, or should not, be able to monopolize certain expensive or rarely needed medical procedures just because they have the means to pay for them. Should states and federal agencies exercise a certain kind of triage by setting a cap on health care expenditures, and then establishing priorities as to who gets what services for what conditions?

I intend to show in this section that individual citizens, including many elderly, can help their own cause and knock the peaks off some of these mountainous expenditures by assuming more and more responsibility for their own health, learning the steps to healing in cases that are not wholly biomechanical, realizing the benefits to be obtained through alternative options, and then helping each other through various educational, developmental, and mutual support activities. The reader should not interpret my descriptions as recommendations or endorsements, but as windows to understanding and doors to other ways of gaining health goals.

# 19. Seniors Helping Themselves

Up to this point, we have considered healing from the standpoint of curing or reversing the course of illness, or enabling people to function in spite of their illnesses. But there's another aspect of healing that needs to be discussed. It is important not only to *make whole* that which has been impaired, but also to *keep whole* what is threatened by life's stresses and traumas. So we should look briefly at the other side of health care—that is, the art of healthy living, especially for seniors.

There is widespread interest in this subject, and a growing number of articles, newsletters, and educational programs aimed at keeping seniors healthier and living longer. There's a substantial element of what I call "the Happy Senior Syndrome," picturing vibrant older people of both sexes quivering with energy and radiating sunshine as they go about their tennis, aerobics classes, and heavy-duty exercise machines. This is great as far as it goes, but one can also recognize an element of self-interest in it for the retirement communities, the insurance companies, and the health food/vitamin sellers who are pushing their own wares as the new-day fountains of youth. But in my own experience, most seniors, like myself, simply want to feel good, live well, and continue to enjoy the things that have always made them happy. To do this, they need simply to transit gracefully from working careers to new careers in retirement, and the main ingredients, from a purely physical standpoint, are the old standards: Diet, rest, and exercise. So a few common-sense remarks about these.

• **Diet:** About a year ago, when I was investigating the problem of medication and the elderly, I wrote a letter to the editor of *Let's Live* magazine, asking readers to send me examples or experiences with mismedication they had learned about. I received replies from ten persons who made a number of valuable suggestions, and seven of these supported alternatives that involved diets or food supplement regimes. Among the respondents were the Nutrition for Optimal Health Association, the Hypoglycemia Association, and the Foundation for Advancements in Science and Education (FASE). Other writers supported methods such as the macrobiotic diet, which features consumption of brown rice and other plant foods balanced and rated on a yin/yang scale; use of large amounts of supplements such as niacin and vitamin C; a number of other natural foods for specific conditions, including trace chromium for fatigue, blue-green algae for general health, a combination anti-oxidant formula to "scavenge" free radicals in the body; and so on.

I know that other organizations such as the American Cancer Society and American Heart Association recommend diets high in certain food groups, like cruciferous vegetables, and avoiding others, such as foods high in cholesterol. Hospitals and health organizations hold meetings and distribute newsletters and recipes dealing with healthy diets. I have no quarrel with any of these, and have no reason to doubt that they will be beneficial to a great majority of senior citizens, but it's hardly necessary to point out that the slogan "One size fits all" hardly applies to any dietary regime.

I've had a couple of experiences that I think have a bearing here. Two or three years before I succeeded in getting off medication with the help of Karen Mahan's computerized biofeedback program, I made another attempt to do so under the guidance of a chiropractor/naturopath who used a dietary approach based on results of tests at an allergy clinic. Under the strictures of this diet, I was to eat no more than two foods per meal for an indefinite period, ostensibly to clear my system of the antibodies that had been produced by a lifetime of eating foods to which I was allergic, at least in some degree. The definition of "food" in terms of this diet included such things as sugar, salt, and other flavorings and additives, so that my meals for four months consisted almost entirely of nuts, fruits, plain cooked grains or vegetables, milk, and a little meat and fish without flavoring or sauces. Anything with corn in it, for example, was verboten. Other foods—rice, liver, and so on—were restricted. Lettuce and tomatoes and a few other things were "free."

At the end of four months, I went back to see the chiropractor. I had lost fifteen pounds and was looking pretty gaunt. My wife had been going crazy trying to cook dinners from the list of allowable foods posted on the refrigerator door. On that visit, the chiropractor opined that enough time had passed to clear my body of the allergies, but he added that he had consulted a couple of cardiologists who had said that because of my age (then seventy), it would be unwise for me to try to stop taking my pills!

To be charitable, I recognized the futility of trying to get off medication by this route, so I went back on a normal diet, soon regained the lost weight, and gave up that particular project.

A bit earlier, I had gone through an effort to replace my pills with GH-3, or Gerovital, the procaine treatment prescribed by the Rumanian doctor-scientist Ana Aslan, who pushed it as a miracle life-extender. I gave the GH-3 plenty of time to get established in my bloodstream, then stopped my medication. The next day I felt positively euphoric for several hours, the best I had felt in years. But one day later, on the golf course, I had played about four holes when I experienced a sinking feeling, a marked weakness, and barely made it back to the clubhouse before climbing into my car and racing home to pop a couple of Tranxene—and I was right back where I started.

As with other lifestyle factors, moderation in all dietary considerations is best. You know what you're most comfortable with, and what gives you problems. Eat moderately what you find enjoyable and beneficial, and avoid foods that you don't. Because older people normally have smaller appetites and eat less than when they were younger, it becomes more important that they eat balanced diets of the things they do need. This is all-important for those who have chronic illnesses such as diabetes that are best controlled by diet. Caregivers and support groups should be concerned that the elderly have the means and encouragement to maintain adequate diets; isolation is one of the worst enemies of those who are not eating adequately, because there is no one around to cheer them up and monitor their eating habits.

• **Rest:** This may not be a major problem for those who have the time and surroundings to enjoy adequate bed rest, but it becomes a factor for those with sleeping disorders, or who "rest" in unhealthy ways. People who lead totally sedentary lives, then spend most of the night prowling around the house or simply lying abed, wide-eyed and worrying, aren't doing much for their bodies, minds, and souls. As in earlier years, the elderly must look for a balance of work, fun, relaxation, and mental activity to attain and maintain optimum vigor for their age.

There are special problems. Many elderly persons continue to work, full-time or part-time, with or without pay. Some of this activity interferes with normal rest. Stimulation associated with work can result in feelings of excitement that make it difficult to sleep, or even to "kick back" and enjoy life without needing to be active all the time.

I can give you a striking example from my own experience. I was editor and part owner of a small monthly newspaper in our community in the early 1980s. Mac, our advertising man, was a wonderful old fellow, then eighty-two, who had more energy than I. How he could make all those contacts and wrestle up all that ad copy every month, I could not imagine, but he did.

One November, however, while he was getting ready for our big Christmas issue, Mac fudged on his rest and sleep, staying up until 1 A.M. on a couple of nights to get his ads done. Immediately afterward, his heart started to act up. He went to see his doctor, who diagnosed "racing heart" or tachycardia. He gave Mac a prescription, and when Mac told me about it, I purposely became visibly upset.

"Mac," I told him, "I'm giving you an order. When you go

home this noon, I want you to go into your bedroom after lunch, close the door, pull down the shades, turn out the light, turn back the bedspread, and *lie down.* Stay there for thirty minutes. Don't try to sleep or do anything else. *Just lie there!* And do it every day from now on!"

Mac listened, gave me a brief nod, and said, "Okay, I'll do it."

When I saw him the next day, his eyes were glistening.

"I did what you told me, and do you know what happened?" he asked.

"No, I don't," I said. "Tell me."

"I lay down and closed my eyes, and woke up an hour and a half later! I felt great!"

He kept up that routine every day for three more years, when he finally played out and died at eighty-five. I don't take any particular credit, but I like to think I helped him to live an active, full life for three more years.

That's all I can really tell you about rest, except that I myself lie down for a half-hour after lunch and dinner every day. It's great for most people after sixty-five or seventy, and it doesn't cost a dime. It's really one of the reasons I retired, because I can remember years in the business world when I'd come back to the office from lunch, look at the pile of junk on my desk, and inwardly lament, "If I could only lie down for fifteen minutes!" Luckily, that ended many years ago, and now I'm realizing what a truly great benefit of retirement it is.

• **Exercise:** The key phrase here is: All your body can tolerate, provided it's something you look forward to and not something you try to avoid. As people grow older they become increasingly aware of their slowly lessening strength and energy. Younger people look at them and wonder why they turn down invitations to evening parties and outdoor expeditions. This is a matter of choice, but there are always three *caveats*: that we not do too much, that we not do too little, and that we do not do the wrong things. I will write further on about double-negative goals, which make it obvious that we need to make *positive* choices. It's an individual call.

If your doctor is not able to give you advice that seems appropriate and congenial to you, there are all kinds of other sources of information and support—hospital programs, county health agencies, your health insurance newsletter, and friends who are attending senior center functions. You are the one affected, you know your own needs and preferences, so you need to make this decision. Whatever your program, treat it as any other goal. Stick with it every day until and unless you make a conscious decision to change it. Patience, perseverance, and determination are as important in reaching this goal as any other.

I've been walking a brisk mile every morning for the past ten years—rain, snow, calm, storm, dark of night, or bright daylight—and it has done wonders for my body tone and mental outlook. My philosophy is that I may have to call on my body in some emergency—a house fire, an automobile accident, or an accident to a loved one—and I want to be able to function without worrying, "This might be bad for my heart!" (Several years ago, I would have thought that, but no longer!) I also do bending and stretching exercises when I get up every morning, and before going to bed at night. This helps me to loosen up and relax. It takes less than five minutes each time, but it lets me know my body is present for duty. It also helps to keep my pulse rate down. If you're bothered by colds, constipation, or other physical nuisances, take a look at how you're exercising (and breathing!).

Those are the basics: diet, rest, and exercise. After that, lifestyles shoot off in all directions. All the experts agree on one thing: Do something! Activities are as varied as humanity itself, and if you can't find something you like, start something of your own.

My brother and I, who were inseparable until I was twenty-one, never lacked for something to do. If we had to kill time while waiting to be picked up from a hike, we'd make up a stupid game, like tossing rocks into a circle in the sand. As long as it was competitive and could be played with any stuff at hand, it was our cup of tea.

There's a sure-fire alternative to games, and it's called *work.* Work is healing. As Voltaire counseled in the closing lines of *Candide,* "Cultivate your garden." Older people know what real work is, probably better than their children and grandchildren. My guess is that any life that is totally devoid of productive work of some kind, be it physical or mental or some combination, is a life without meaning. Work that involves doing for others always has compensations, whether in-kind, financial, or emotional.

Elders can often repay their children and others with such chores as baby-sitting their grandchildren, house-sitting for neighbors, taking in newspapers or mail during others' vacations, tutoring, checking homework, telling stories (including their own experiences), taking phone calls or writing letters, and so on. If you can't find anything on your own hook, call your nearest church, school, or library and ask. Better get ready for some real challenges!

While I was writing this, I read an article in *Longevity* magazine (February 1991) that told about a community-wide program to reduce the risk of heart disease. This was conducted in Monterey and Salinas, California, in 1980 by Stanford University's Center for Research in Disease Prevention. The education-centered effort had the goal of getting the 120,000 residents to stop smoking, eat less fat and more fruits and vegetables, control their weight and blood pressure, and exercise—in other words, to adopt a lifestyle that would promote better health and increased longevity. The public education phase ended in 1986, and since then the researchers have been evaluating their data. The results, recently published, can be summed up: Community-wide health education works!

Educational messages in mass media averaged 527 per year during the campaign. Five years after the campaign ended, most of the programs were still in place and functioning. Businesses cooperated by having aerobic exercise periods for their employees. One thousand people pledged to stop smoking. Mass mailings backed up the media campaign. Many housewives were attracted by the gourmet quality of the health recipes provided.

The most dramatic statistic showed a thirteen percent decline in smoking. There was an average drop of 1 percent in cholesterol, 4 percent in blood pressure, and 3 percent in resting pulse

THE ART OF HEALING

rate.

One doctor who co-directed the project pointed out that, if the two percent decline in cholesterol were extended across the country, it could save 30,000 lives a year. The success was so striking that similar campaigns have been funded in Pawtucket, R.I.; Mankato and Bloomington, Minn.; and Fargo-Moorhead on the North Dakota-Minnesota border. This is something seniors could work on in their own communities.

Safety is always a concern. Senior citizens have hazards in their homes that might not threaten younger people, such as slippery bathtubs or uneven carpets. I suggest that caregivers and counselors make a safety inventory of their clients' homes to remove or neutralize anything that might cause accidents. Information is available on making homes more livable for elders by placing light switches and cabinets within reach, lowering key work spaces, dividing stored "keepables" into lighter loads, and so on.

An important note: The Environmental Protection Agency recently published a study showing that indoor pollution may be a greater health hazard than previously thought. The agency examined 600 homes in northern New Jersey and Los Angeles, and found pollution inside people's homes to be worse than outside. Chloroform, probably resulting from chlorine released from hot water during showers, was one of the pollutants discovered. Another was benzene, the main source suspected being cigarette smoke.

All the foregoing applies to older peoples' micro-environments—those things that relate to their houses and their immediate surroundings. But they and their caregivers should always be aware of the more general environmental setting. Here are a few things to be aware of:

• **Weather-related problems:** Almost every climate will have an adverse impact on human beings at some time of year. Older people are more sensitive to extremes of heat and cold, and suffer health problems sooner. Heating and cooling systems should be functional, easily adjusted, and given maintenance checks annually. Some older people have a strong inclination to pinch pennies and put on more sweaters when it gets too cold, or simply suffer from the heat in the summer. Someone should visit their homes from time to time, at different times of day and year, to guard against this. It's also a good argument for having live-in help, at least on a part-time basis. Flu shots are recommended for the elderly in advance of the flu season.

• **Traffic:** This can impact anyone, but the elderly are more susceptible because there is no escape for them if they are confined to their homes. Traffic noise may interfere with sleep, fast-moving vehicles are dangerous on streets that are too wide for the elderly to cross safely, or the house may be inconvenient to public transportation. This is an important consideration when the time comes to decide where the elderly client is going to live.

• **Electromagnetic radiation and low frequency sound:** These factors can cause headaches, nervousness, rapid pulse, and loss of sleep without being suspected. Electrical technicians and sound engineers can sometimes point a finger at possible sources of these nuisances, but utilities are often loath to make suggestions or recommendations because they resist accepting responsibility for such problems. If you can find an objective professor of environmental health, or even a TV technician with a spectrum analyzer, you may be able to get a reading on such problems.

• **Neighborhood factors:** The social environment is often unhealthy for older people. Large numbers continue to live in the homes they have occupied for decades while the neighborhoods around these homes deteriorate through lack of maintenance, neglect of streets, lighting, and other elements of the infrastructure. It may be hard to persuade the older person to move, but that may be the only answer to allay the fear and disgust they feel because of littered and overgrown yards, vandalism, frequent fights and disturbances, late-night noises, or even pistol shots and auto crashes. This is a problem of communities, not just individuals, but it is often beyond the point where the older residents themselves can do much about it.

There are positive aspects of the environment, of course, but these are usually the things one is moving toward, not away from. Such are retirement communities with amenities already

provided; new neighborhoods to which friends or relatives have
already moved; smaller and more convenient houses or apart-
ments on one level, without stairs, where the needs of everyday
living are conveniently at hand. A third-party peer counselor
may be the type of person best able to assess the needs of the
elderly clients and persuade them to take the steps that will
make them happier and more secure.

While this is not a treatise on human psychology, we should
not leave this chapter on healing the ills of the elderly, and
helping them to a greater share of life's satisfactions, without
summing up the attitudes and practices on their part that are
most likely to make these things happen. From my own experience, these are the most significant:

1. **Set positive goals:** This is essential for anyone, but especially
   for the retired elderly, if they are to stay healthy and optimistic. An example of a good short-range goal might be to read a
   book such as *The Power of Positive Thinking* by Dr. Norman
   Vincent Peale, within the following three months. A longer-
   term goal might be to get together with your children and
   decide how your life's possessions are to be divided following your death. Nearly everyone I know wants to be in
   control of this process, but few have the ambition and self-
   discipline actually to organize it and carry it out. You can't
   keep your mind off your troubles without having positive
   goals to think about.

2. **Communicate:** Phone, write, or visit your loved ones and
   others on your Christmas card list as frequently as common
   sense and your budget allow. Buy a roll of stamps and give
   yourself a time limit for using them up. Ask for writing paper
   and envelopes as presents, or buy them yourself. Frequent
   short communications are better than long ones. Try to be
   interesting, and *always* ask questions that elicit a response.
   Keep your opinions about the tastes and actions of others to
   yourself. Judge not, lest ye be judged!

3. **Work and serve:** If you're able, volunteer to help with the
   activities of your church, your service club or social group,
   your senior center or your schools. Many groups such as
   RSVP (Retired Senior Volunteer Program) are tailor-made for

seniors who want to work with younger people at their own pace in areas of their own interest. Activity like this helps you to feel *good* whether you feel *well* or not.

4. **Do everything you can for yourself:** If you want to stay in your home and be independent, don't expect your neighbors and children to be coming over all the time to do little things for you. But if they do, simply thank them; don't complain about how hard things are for you. If your spouse is living, help each other to be independent. It may sound hard-boiled, but don't spoil your spouse just because you want to appear gallant or tender-hearted. If you do, you may become co-dependents very rapidly.

5. **Settle your affairs:** Write things down, make lists, pick a funeral plan and arrange to finance it. Don't leave things dangling just because you're too tired, or "can't think about that just now."

6. **If you were ever a Boy Scout**, reaffirm your Scout oath: "On my honor, I will do my best to do my duty to God and my country and to obey the Scout law; to help other people at all times, and to keep myself physically fit, mentally awake, and morally straight." This requires you to obey the Scout law, which says that a Scout is trustworthy, loyal, friendly, kind, helpful, courteous, cheerful, obedient, thrifty, brave, clean, and reverent. If you are all of those things still, you're okay.

7. **Be a friend:** If you're alone, try to make a pal of someone you like, someone you can drop in on (or vice versa) for coffee or shopping or just a talk; someone to play golf and bridge with, or to bum around with. When you have such a pal, you're never alone! (It could even be a dog or cat!)

# 20. The Art of Healing

We have just considered some of the things seniors can do for themselves to get healthy and to stay healthy. But there still remain all the factors that cause or contribute to illnesses of all kinds, and these must be addressed for those of us (including myself) who need the help of professionals to address them successfully. In the first two parts of this book, I discussed the structural aspects of our health care system that make this process maddeningly difficult and, in too many cases, barely possible.

One of the most pressing of these problems is our prevailing medical model, which dictates that the doctor diagnose and treat his patients. This is done on the basis of examinations and tests that measure symptoms that can be determined or verified by readouts accessible to the five senses—sight, hearing, touch, taste, or smell. Thus, the patient's temperature is 102 degrees, some 3 degrees above normal; the blood sugar is 240, or 90 points above the top of the normal range; blood pressure is 160/105, well above the desirable 120/80; the PSA (prostatic specific antigen) is 8.3 versus a desirable 4.0 or less; and so on.

It really comes down to the difference between treating and healing, as I have suggested. I have discussed the now-prevalent biomechanical treatment model in the preceding pages. I shall define and discuss the healing model in those that follow. The difference between the two models is well expressed in this aphorism: "Give a man a pill, and you have cured his illness. Teach him how to be well, and you have given him a new life."

Healing is making whole. It is restoring an organism to its normal, healthy, fully functioning self. Health means wholeness; the two words are the same. They refer to the soundness and vigor of the whole person—body, mind, and spirit. I shall have more to say about the spiritual aspect of health in Part IV.

For the most part, people heal themselves. Left alone, through common sense and the experience of past illnesses, people get well without further intervention in a great majority of cases. The processes, which have been exhaustively researched for decades, are well known: a nourishing diet, plenty of rest, freedom from demands for too much physical work and emotional stress—and time. Time is truly the great healer, but that fact is overlooked in the mad scramble for instant relief. "Fast, fast, fast relief—starts working in just seven seconds," say the commercials, and people buy the product, because they don't want to wait eight seconds for their pills to start "working."

When we think of true healing, as distinct from our biomedical models, we should first look at the critical forces involved. A few key words will serve us well in this connection. They are LOVE, INTEGRATION, BELIEF, HOPE, ATTITUDE, SUPPORT, and TIME.

The first of these is love. Not just love in the sense meant by the teenager who writes to Dear Abby: "How can I tell whether I'm in love or not?" But love in the sense of the unselfish other-directedness the mother feels for her baby, that old friends hold for each other, that soldiers feel for their foxhole buddies, for whom they would die before letting them down. This is the most important healing force of all, and I'll have much to say about it.

The second is integration. When people say they're falling apart, they're not kidding; the truth is that they're suffering from disintegration of body, mind, and spirit. Reintegrating them is simply making whole or healthy again, but it is more than putting parts back together. It is putting those parts together in the right way, in the right order, and at the right time. This requires knowledge and understanding rather than plain skill, although skill is needed in the actual work of reassembly. Examples are plentiful—the man who has lost his motivation for working because his wife has left him; the woman whose child has run away from home; parents whose teenager has committed suicide; the middle-aged manager whose employer has closed up shop. These folks need some kind of counseling or support to put their lives, their minds, their bodies back together.

The key words for patients are belief, hope, and attitude—first, belief that they have the power to heal themselves; second, hope that success is certain if they have the motivation, courage, and persistence to do it; and finally, attitude. They either have a positive attitude, that they are going to get well and nothing can stop them; or a negative attitude, that there is nothing on earth that can make them well.

Another key is support. Healing can be a slow, difficult, and perhaps failing business if there are no family members or friends around to keep the atmosphere cheerful and optimistic. Support groups including others sharing the same problems are invaluable, for the same reasons.

And, of course, time. Learning patience, to wait for healing to take place at its own proper pace, is difficult for most people. But this is exactly when love, belief, hope, and support are most needed.

There are many splendid books on this subject, some of which are listed in the bibliography at the back of this book. The one that comes to mind first is *Love, Medicine and Miracles* by Dr. Bernie Siegel. It is tempting simply to copy great stretches of the book in this space, and there wouldn't be much left to say. However, because his theme is only part of this story, I must refer to his major emphases here, and urge that you find this book and read it.

A cancer surgeon himself, Dr. Siegel came to his understanding of the processes of disease, and of healing, only through long and rigorous experience with patients suffering from all types of tumors and with all kinds of outcomes. One of his first discoveries was that he could not begin to provide sympathetic treatment and support for his patients until he learned how to listen to them and to understand their illnesses. This took into account their personalities, their work, their home life, and social activities.

He points out that treating cancer involves a two-person team, the doctor and the patient. He says, "The best results proceed from a 'negotiation' in which the practitioner's view-point and that of the patient come close enough together for true communication. . . . To me the true measure of wholistic medi-cine is how well the patient and the doctor accept each other's belief system, even though their beliefs may differ. Neither one of us forces something on the other."

Following chapters on the role of the mind in disease and healing, the use of visualization and other methods (which will be discussed under modalities), Dr. Siegel comes to his views on the critical role of love. He writes: "When we choose to love, healing energy is released in the body. Energy itself is loving and intelligent and available to all of us."

This comports precisely with my own experiential perception, which is that love is the gravity of the spirit universe. It is what binds everything together. Note that Dr. Siegel and I are saying the same thing: Love is real. It is energy, or a force similar to gravity that can have miraculous results when focused by the mind and spirit on human targets such as cancer. (Perhaps prayer has a role in this, and vice versa.)

The essence of love is in giving, and giving unconditionally. If one loves another only in the expectation of return, one will be disappointed, because what is returned is often not what the lover expected. And there may be no return at all, at least to the immediate senses; but love heals the giver as well as the recip-ient, so when it is given unconditionally, it will be returned in full measure from another source. As James Russell Lowell wrote, "Who gives of himself with his gift feeds three: Himself, his hungering neighbor, and Me."

How does love heal? I am convinced that what love does is to fill our hearts and minds and bodies so completely that there is no room left for illness to operate—illness, or any other negative aspects of our lives, especially fear. Or the effects of stress, which can be all-encompassing and all-consuming.

Stress-induced fear can produce panic attacks, which make one feel that an evil entity has him by the windpipe and is choking off the air from his lungs, while another entity is tying his stomach into knots. I've been there, and that's about as close as I can come to a description.

There is an inescapable linkage between love and fear that has been expressed in many ways, by many writers, some of the best-known examples being in the Bible.

- Perfect love casteth out fear.
- Greater love hath no man than this, that he give his life for his friend.
- Of what, then, art thou afraid? If God be with thee, who can be against thee?
- Fear not, for lo, I am with thee alway.

And as I indicated earlier, love is the true force that sends soldiers into battle to get the job done for their buddies.

In its bearing on healing, I have formulated the syllogism this way:

Love is liberating.
If love frees us from fear, love also enables us to heal ourselves.
Fear lies behind our failure to cope with stress, and healing cannot take place in the presence of stress.
If love banishes fear, and freedom from fear allows us to cope with stress, love therefore enables healing to take place.
And only when we are fully healed are we fully free.

This perception was reinforced in a beautiful letter that I received from Dr. Jerry Jampolsky, director of the Center for Attitudinal Healing in Tiburon, California. I was researching the problem of overmedication of the elderly, and asked him if there was any connection between fear and addiction. His reply:

Fear is what makes us want to keep separate from others, from ourselves, and from God. Our egos would have us create gods of our own making, in order to keep away from

God and each other. This causes us to become attached to things—chocolates, phenobarbital, smoking, heroin, crack, and so on, which are being used as a substitute for love in our relationships.

The pain which results is caused by guilt and fear. It causes us to seek things to relieve our suffering. The way we suffer is a feeling of emptiness inside because the ego covers up the fact that we have all the love there is in the world—the love of God, which is always inside us.

What happens when we learn to trust in God is that we feel totally loved and our addictive needs can then begin to disappear.

When we realize gradually that the love of God is our essence and that all we need to do to be happy is to accept that happiness and joy, and give that away to others unconditionally, we find that we don't really need anything from anyone else.

I became acquainted with the important work of Dr. Jampolsky when I read his book *Teach Only Love.* In his introduction, Dr. Jampolsky sets out his theme in a powerful, lucid fashion.

As we emerge from the birth canal, we enter the world desperately struggling for breath. Most of us travel through life continuing to struggle, feeling unloved and alone. All too often we are afraid. Afraid of sickness and death, afraid of God, even afraid of continuing to live. Often we leave the world the same way we entered it—desperately struggling for breath.

I believe there is another way of looking at life that makes it possible for us to walk through the world in love, at peace, and without fear. This other way requires no external battles, but only that we heal ourselves. It is a process I call "attitudinal healing," because it is internal and primarily a mental process. Properly practiced, it will, I believe, allow anyone, regardless of his circumstances, to begin experiencing the joy and harmony each instant contains, and to start his journey on a path of love and hope.

The mind can be retrained. Within this fact lies our freedom. No matter how often we have misused it, the mind can be utilized in a way that is so positive that at first it is beyond anything we can imagine.

Dr. Jampolsky has put these principles into practice by opening and directing his healing center in Tiburon. Near the beginning of the book he writes:

As a doctor, I believed that gentleness and empathy were nice attributes to have, but that it was not absolutely necessary for the practice of love and the practice of medicine to go hand in hand. I came to see that healing and love are inseparable, and so I wanted our center to be a place where every attempt that anyone made to help himself or another would be thoroughly gentle and completely kind.

There is much more that is extremely insightful and uplifting for anyone engaged in the healing arts, but as with Dr. Siegel's book, you have to read it all to get its full import and flavor. He points out that the use of his methods is not limited to children and adults with catastrophic illnesses, but also has application for everyone.

It is really startling to me how my experiences and those of others I have interviewed are cross-validated at every turn. Thus Karen Mahan, my own mentor and therapist, says this about drugs and fear:

There is *always* a fear behind drug dependency. The stresses have triggered the body to symptomize (a neat way of saying, "get sick") and the symptoms trigger fear. This is either the fear of death, or of becoming non-functional. The subject *already* can't handle what he has got (in the way of stresses) before the symptoms appear. The body makes that clear; that's why the symptoms show up. The body says, "You may die, or become totally disabled."

So what do people do? They take the drugs that buffer their symptoms. If the person is so overtaxed that the demands are too heavy for his body, he is set up for pills. But even with the pills, the stress still prevents healing.

In very few cases of older people on drugs is the fear not already there. It may be an initial reaction, which can be appropriate, but as time goes on and the situation changes, it can be inappropriate. Many people simply *drug their fear,* thus getting farther away from reality.

Does it sound to you that Karen Mahan and Dr. Jampolsky are reading off the same page? Of course it does, because they are both reading from the Book of Reality. Anyone else who reads this book will find the same words.

Karen goes on to discuss her way of dealing with this, a paradigm of caring commitment, which produces results—that is, progressive changes in her clients, a dissipation of the symptoms, the identification and disposal of root causes—and along with the process, the evaporation of fear. The client also identifies and classifies his own personal goals toward which he will work in a positive way—in other words, to work toward an end result that is his deepest wish. The client is hardly aware of this as it is happening, but every so often will open his eyes wide, burst out laughing or crying, and Karen will exclaim, "Aha!" She adds, "People think they can't confront their phobias, but they can, and I show them how."

Larry Feldman, a California rehabilitation counselor, wrote a fine little book entitled *Feeling Better.* He writes:

No matter what your condition, there is always something you can do to feel better. Healing and recovery are directly related to our mood, attitude and stress level. I point out [to my patients] not only the importance of hope and a positive outlook, but how you can change your outlook to bring about positive results in any pain and physical condition.

Stress may not cause your pain or your inability to function, but can so rob your body of vitality and energy that healing cannot take place. . . . The stress of chronic pain and inability to function are major barriers to recovery, and you can learn to free the energy that is wasted in stress and tension.

Do you see a vicious circle here? It's the real Catch-22 of stress-related illnesses, which *all* have a psychosomatic dimension. Stress causes many symptoms including pain and loss of function; and as Feldman states above, chronic pain and inability to function can cause new stresses, which hinder recovery. So you are left to find a person or method, such as Karen Mahan's, which can sidetrack the Stress Express and clear your path to the Recovery Shortline.

A key to persuading seniors to get help for their problems is the expression of concern by family members and friends. Jean Dunlop, who designed the Addictions Treatment Services Program for Older Adults at St. Vincent Hospital in Portland, says:

> Treatment is personalized and stresses family participation. One family member, or two at most, should—in a real supportive way—tell the person that they care about them and want them to get help. Too many times I've seen patients who were confronted by the entire family. That just makes·them feel shame.

A recent study of sixty-nine men and women aged forty-eight to seventy-five, conducted by Dr. Karen Altergott of Purdue University, showed that those with active, mutually supportive relationships often continue to live high-quality lives. The people in that group had been recently diagnosed as having cancer. One-third of them developed serious depression and the other two-thirds did not. What made the difference?

A sentence in an article in *Modern Maturity* magazine, reporting the results of this study, provided an explanation:

> They [those who did not develop depression] sought information from community resources or publications that helped them deal with their illness; they had a sense of usefulness, not dependence; and they had frequent contact with close friends with whom they were completely open about their condition.

It would be interesting to know what the outcomes of the two groups' illnesses turned out to be, but all research would give the socially supported group a far higher chance for remission.

There are thousands of practitioners of the healing arts who place a loving commitment to their clients above financial rewards to themselves. One of these is Dr. M. Scott Peck, a psychiatrist and author of *The Road Less Traveled* and *People of the Lie.* In the latter book, he reports an interesting case of a client who resisted every attempt on his part to get to the bottom of her personal problems so he could begin her healing. After some two years of frequent sessions at $75 each, she told him she was going to have to give up her treatments, saying she thought she was getting nowhere. He explained patiently that she had not been giving him full cooperation, but that he would keep working with her for as long as she wanted.

"But this has been very expensive for me," she said, "and besides, I know you wouldn't want to continue seeing me if I couldn't pay you."

Peck had to think only a few moments before telling her, "Charlene, I have real affection for you and want to see you well and happy. Money is not the only reason I'm working with you. If it will help you, I'll continue to treat you for half the regular fee."

One by one, Peck overcame her defenses until she felt compelled to continue treatment. The ending was not completely happy, as Charlene's problems remained unresolved after long treatment; but at least, Peck's declaration of a loving commitment opened the door to healing, and it was no fault of his that Charlene was not able to walk through it.

Most of what we have said about love and healing applies to people of all ages, but there is a special problem for the elderly— the fear of death. Because this deals finally with the problems of spirituality, of existence and eternity, we shall defer a full consideration of it until the next chapter. But because we have talked about the other fears here, we should address the issue insofar as it concerns the care teams, the families, and others involved with the healing process. This is because the most important healing of all is that which involves the final healing or cleansing of the spirit before it leaves the body and its earthly home. Those connected with the care of the terminally ill, and with it the hospice function, should at least be aware of the process.

I think that all those who approach death, especially through illness, should be guided to think about their unfinished business on earth before they walk through that door. The moments before death will likely be the most traumatic of a person's experience unless this groundwork has been laid. I am a strong proponent of mentally rehearsing death before it becomes imminent, and those who help to initiate this process must possess a special delicacy, authority, and unswerving commitment, or they may well be turned off short of the goal. The purpose should be to put the patient's mind as completely at ease as far ahead of the final hour as possible. Discretion, privacy, and plenty of time will be required. The pain and symptomology of bodily illness become irrelevant. I think it is a gross disservice to the elderly ill to zonk them out with drugs in the moments just prior to their passing. They should be allowed to be lucid, to recognize those around them, to express any final thoughts, and to be alert as the moment arrives.

I think of a dear sister-in-law, a resident of Phoenix, Arizona, who lay dying with her husband at her bedside. He phoned us in King City, Oregon, only ten minutes after she passed on, and said with wonder in his voice,

"Helen Marie just looked up at me and asked, 'How am I supposed to do this?' Then she was gone."

That is the way it should be—clear minds and clear communications until the end.

This shouldn't be a time of dread, of fear, of cries for forgiveness and confession. It should be, so far as possible, a time of quiet reflection, of simple communication, of hand squeezes and hugs and smiles and tears, and it may be that the only words necessary will be, "I love you" and "God bless you." There should be no exclusions or rancor or jealousy, or feelings of "Who's closest to her?" or "Who should or shouldn't be here?" at this time—the only dictum being that the wishes of the patient should be scrupulously respected. We shall leave a more philosophical discussion for the next chapter.

We shall also leave until later a substantive discussion of the mind in healing. This is necessary because of a long history of confusion between the entities called mind and spirit; whether they are just one entity, or if two, which has dominance over the other. Most writing with a psychological approach in recent decades has used the term "mind" to include both mind and spirit, and I think this has caused a lot of confusion and misunderstanding.

But even more significant, in my opinion, are recent trends toward unifying spirituality and hard sciences in the fields of astrophysics and cosmology, which will have decisive effects on the direction of medicine and health care. I prefer to leave a discussion of these trends, also, to Part IV, and at this point simply mention that the mind and body are equally involved in what I have written thus far, as well as in the comments that follow.

# 21. Healing Modalities

I think this is the place to talk about the various "soft" methodologies that are available to supplement, or, with caution, to replace the biomedical practices that doctors generally follow. I must assert caution in this connection, because there will be argument about whether any of the "biomechanical" methods can or should actually be replaced; but the possibility must be considered, because if the patient can be healed before it is necessary to see a doctor, then that door should be left open so long as all parties know what is going on.

It will help to think about these methodologies in the context of the so-called "holistic" (or "wholistic") model, which has been in the public eye for several decades. This is, briefly, an attempt, or movement, to bring all the healing professions into one concert, to enable the patient to have access to all the expertise, agencies, and methodologies that may be best for his particular needs. The preface of a book entitled *Health for the Whole Person* describes it this way:

> In our discussions among ourselves and with the contributing authors we defined three aspects of a holistic approach. First, such an approach involves expanding our focus to include the many personal, familial, social and environmental factors that promote health, prevent illness, and encourage healing. Second, a holistic approach views the

patient as an individual person, not as a symptom-bearing organism. This attitude emphasizes the self-responsibility of the person for his or her health and the importance of mobilizing the person's own health capacities, rather than treating illness only from the outside. Third, the holistic approach tries to make wise use of the many diagnostic, treatment, and health modalities that are available in addition to the standard *materia medica*—including alternative medical and healing systems as well as psychological techniques and physical modalities.

The biomechanical methods include all the usual treatments you expect to get when you go to a doctor, such as surgery, prescription medication, physical therapy, and the standard lectures on diet, rest, and exercise. Institutional care in hospitals, skilled nursing facilities, sanitaria, and the like are also in this category.

The "soft" methodologies have been widely discussed in the public and special-group media in recent years, and anyone seeking detailed information can usually obtain it from any of the professional groups and non-profit educational associations that deal with each method. I'll name and describe the principal modalities and indicate how I think they fit into the overall health picture.

It's important to point out that many of these modalities are unfamiliar to some if not most seniors, as their acceptance has generally been among the younger patient groups, or associated with good health practices unrelated to illness. Biofeedback would be an example of this; it did not come into general use until the 1970s, and even now has not been experienced by many older Americans.

But in moving from a biomechanical mode of health care to a more open style, or even a combination, as many peer counselors may urge their clients to do, one has to take into account that an important task of persuasion must be undertaken: first, to convince the client that it is both safe and desirable to try some alternative style of care; and second, that this particular style is the one with the greatest potential benefit. This is an overriding reason why the peer counselor, of an age and experience at least matching the client's, is the person best suited to do this. I should also note that there is wide variation in the relative degree of acceptance of these modalities by the medical profession, with some, such as psychotherapy, being generally approved, while others, such as acupuncture, may be viewed with skepticism if not hostility.

So let us look at some of the more common methods:

• **Psychology and psychotherapy.** This involves professional psychologists, usually with Ph.D. degrees, who counsel clients, try to identify their problems, and arrive at insights that enable the clients, with guidance and continued probing, to change their ways of thinking, and thus their lives for the better. Peer counselors can play an important role in convincing elderly clients that such counseling does not hint at mental illness on their part, but that, on the contrary, it will help to clarify their thinking and simplify their self-management.

The importance of this branch of healing is made clear by Gene D. Cohen in his book *The Brain in Human Aging*:

> Given the prevalence of somatic (bodily) illness in later life, one is more likely to find a greater interplay of mental and physical disorders in the elderly as compared to other age groups; that is, mental illness is less likely to occur in isolation in older adults than in younger ones. . . . Here we confront one of the most important "sleepers" on the public health front—the impact of psychological state and mental status on the course of overall health and illness in later life, the influence of psyche (mind) on soma (body) with aging.

The writer gives an example of this assertion:

> In a now classic study by Levitan and Kornfeld (1981) the investigators compared the clinical outcomes of two groups of elderly patients who underwent surgery for fractured femurs. The treatment group of twenty-four patients aged sixty-five and older received psychiatric consultation during hospitalization, while the control group of twenty-six

patients in the same age group did not receive any psychiatric intervention. The groups were alike in terms of reason for admission (a broken thigh bone), age, surgical intervention, hospital setting and overall medical care—except that one group received psychiatric consultation while the other group did not. The group receiving psychiatric attention revealed two major outcome differences from the control group. The treatment group had (1) a substantially shorter length of stay in the hospital, and (2) a significantly improved clinical outcome.

We must alert the reader that health professionals make a distinction between the work of psychiatrists, who are medical doctors following the model of diagnosis and treatment, and psychologists, who do not have medical degrees. They are both working with the human mind and brain, but the educational emphasis is quite different, the psychiatrists having the full medical school training in addition to their schooling as specialists, while psychologists' studies place less emphasis on the physical basis of mental processes.

The various schools of thought in psychology, and the specific techniques they use, are of less significance than their goals, which are to access the non-physical causes of a patient's problems through verbal consultations and testing, and to bring his thinking into line with the realities of his actual life situation. Opening the door to a great variety of options, and restructuring the patient's perception of himself relative to those realities, are key steps in the process.

Virtually all psychologists accept the need for a multidisciplinary approach to uncover the patient's physical, emotional, mental, and personality disorders, such as dysthymia, which is a depressive neurosis. Free association, the Rohrshach (blot) tests, art therapy as a diagnostic and therapeutic tool, confrontation therapy, and group therapy are just a few of the dozens of methods that may be used by individual psychologists.

• **Relaxation therapy.** This follows several different approaches, some perhaps meriting separate discussion, but all have the aim of calming the mind and, through it, the body, or vice versa. In my experience, it is difficult to quiet the mind for any extended period just through bodily relaxation, unless it is ready to be quieted. On the other hand, once the mind is at rest, or focused on restful things, bodily relaxation often follows. This assumes that a restful, comfortable position is maintained.

Some of the better known techniques, in which relaxation may be a primary or secondary goal, are:

• **Meditation.** This covers a variety of practices, all of which have a goal of mental and physical relaxation and openness to any ideas that enter the mind, without being forced. Transcendental meditation, for example, follows a structured routine of daily observances of a quiet period, uncluttered surroundings, and no interference from any external source. It is important that this last for an adequate period—usually at least an hour—once a day. Dr. Pelletier, in his book cited earlier, says this:

> The fundamental process of meditation . . . is to gain *mastery over attention.* The goal of this mastery is to "develop an awareness which allows every stimulus to enter into consciousness devoid of our normal selection process, devoid of normal tuning or input selection of model building and devoid of normal categorizing" (quoting Naranjo and Ornstein, 1971). The meditator stops his ordinary cognitive processes so as to experience direct perception of stimuli, devoid of preconception.

I would describe this process as the passive opening of the mind and spirit to any external messages that they may be prepared to receive.

The payoff from meditation that is not available from some of the other practices is the stimulation of perceptions not previously recognized. The sources of these perceptions, whether from supernatural sources, "cultural memory," or other agency, may be subject to debate, but the fact that they occur is not.

• **Visualization.** This is a specific form of meditation that follows a different pattern of recommended steps. The rationale for visualization is that positive images called up in the mind, relating to a specific situation or physical condition (such as cancer) can have a powerful effect on how the body and its immune system respond to the threat. Dr. O. Carl Simonton, in his landmark book *Getting Well Again,* reported great success with patients who were taught to visualize their immune organisms attacking the cancers at the source and progressively diminishing them. He had each patient draw diagrams as to how he or she pictured this mentally, and while the diagrams differed considerably, the impact on the progress of the disease was remarkably consistent.

Dr. Siegel thought that images of attacking the disease may work for about 20 percent of the patients, but that 80 percent need a different approach to heal. The use of imagery and reducing it to pictures drawn by the patients proved more useful than laboratory tests in assessing the patients' prospects, according to work done by the Simontons, Jeanne Achterberg, and G. Frank Lawlis, who concluded, "The blood chemistries offer information only about the current state of the disease, whereas psychological variables offer future insights."

Visualization has many other uses, probably because it is an important factor in maintaining a positive attitude and influencing desirable outcomes in various situations. (Psychologists will tell you this is not limited to health applications; it has equal force in virtually any human activity, such as sports competition, sales presentations, maybe even proposing to the girl of your dreams. If you visualize a good result, you gain confidence, and are more likely to act in such a way as to bring it about.)

• **Autogenics.** This is a form of relaxation therapy that depends on the subject's success, when in a state of self-hypnosis, or inward-directed consciousness, in imagining the limbs becoming heavy and the flesh and organs becoming warm. This "controlled feeling" routine has the purpose of creating the same dilation of blood vessels and capillaries, and the same slackness of the limbs and large muscles, that are the end products of other forms of relaxation. You might think of it as relaxation in reverse; that is, beginning with the result of other kinds of exercise, and moving backward to the controlling mechanisms such as the mind and nervous stimuli. Properly learned and applied, it is a very effective method.

Some other relaxation techniques, such as the Jacobson method, use similar principles and achieve much the same results.

• **Biofeedback.** This is a discipline that encompasses a number of sub-modalities, each with its own techniques and uses. Briefly, it is the use of playback instruments and signals that help one learn how to regulate autonomic or unconsciously directed systems, such as blood pressure or skin temperature, in an intentional, consistent way. There are instruments that are attached to different parts of the body and that give continuous readouts by gauges, buzzers, or tones. By noting the changes in these signals, one learns to make muscles relax, or skin temperature to rise, just by the way one senses his or her own feelings. The principal instruments are these:

*Electromyograph.* This responds to changes in electrical currents through a muscle or muscle groups, in increments of microvolts. The lower the reading, the more relaxed the muscle.

*Thermistor.* This reads skin temperature at the surface (for example, the tip of the index finger), and usually registers in degrees Fahrenheit. The fingertips are one of the easier places for most people to warm. Other parts of the body, such as the ankles or toes, may be more difficult, but with practice can be made warmer, and this has more overall benefit as one becomes able to transfer the warming to larger areas of the body. When muscles and nerves are thoroughly relaxed, the blood flows more freely and all parts of the body, including the skin, tend to reach a balanced temperature.

*Galvanic skin response (GSR).* This is the same as the lie detector, as it senses an increase in the conductivity of the skin because of the presence of moisture. Under the pressure of mental stress, the skin tends to perspire more, and this raises the skin's conductivity. This is a very sensitive instrument, and a lot of experience is required to evaluate its results, as an increase in conductivity can be due to causes other than lying.

*Electroencephalograph (EEG).* This is the instrument that monitors brain waves, displaying them on a scale of cycles (waves) per second. The intensity or "size" of the waves is also indicated. The significance of this is that the lower the frequency, the calmer the brain (or mind) is. Activity in this regard ranges from deep sleep on the lower end of the scale to great excitement or emotional activity on the high end. With practice, those being monitored can learn to induce a tranquil alpha frequency by concentrating on pleasant, peaceful thoughts, and this in turn reduces the activity of most of the body's organs.

*Combined readouts.* I was lucky enough to work with a computer-linked biofeedback instrumentation that showed my pulse rate, the depth of upper chest breathing, and abdominal breathing in separate lines, simultaneously, on a TV-type screen. This enabled me to learn how to slow my pulse in order to establish an idealized RSA (Respiratory Sinus Arrhythmia), which is the characteristic slowing of the heartbeat at a consistent point in the exhalation phase of proper breathing. You really don't know whether you are breathing properly until you have seen your own lung/heart rhythm on such an instrument. That was what enabled me to get off prescription drugs, as I became competent to overcome the tachycardia (fast pulse) that had torpedoed past efforts to quit.

- **Alternative medical treatments.** This category includes doctors with degrees other than medical doctors, dentists, and certain specialists, and includes chiropractors, naturopaths, osteopaths, and homeopaths. Many practitioners hold doctorates in more than one of these disciplines.

*Chiropractic* confines itself largely to the diagnosis and treatment of subluxations of the spine, which are misalignments of the vertebrae relative to the other vertebrae in the spinal column. The aim is to permit the unimpeded operation of the central nervous system, which depends heavily on the column of nerves that passes along the spine and sends branching nerves to the limbs and organs. Many chiropractors also prescribe exercise and diet regimes to promote good health, and may include such modalities as acupuncture, massage, and homeopathy in their practice.

*Osteopathy* is similar to chiropractic in its principles and healing aims, but focuses on the importance of unimpeded circulation. Osteopaths work with the skeletal structure and musculature in their treatments, but many have come to regard the techniques of manipulation as secondary to medication and surgery.

*Homeopathy* is based on the belief that symptoms of illness are best treated by agents that tend to produce the same symptoms in the patient. For example, diarrhea might be treated by giving the patient a very small dose of a laxative. The idea is that the body's own healing powers and immune system will react against the introduction of a new symptom-creating agent and, in fighting it, will abate the other symptom as well.

*Naturopathy* attempts to use natural forces to maintain health and treat disease. Typical remedies include sun-bathing, diet regimes, steam bathing, exercise, and manipulations. High vegetable consumption is encouraged as is abstinence from salt and stimulants.

All the above four disciplines may also include reliance on natural remedies such as herbs, oils, flower extracts, and the like, and may also borrow from, or lean on, crystallography, reflexology, iridology, health food supplements such as vitamins and minerals, and so on. Physiotherapy is also important to them, and is used as a supplementary treatment or by referral for specific conditions, such as muscle tension, and for retraining muscles and healing injuries. There seem to be few hard-and-fast lines of distinction between the various disciplines any more, and even medical doctors disagree as to which kinds of treatment may be useful and acceptable, and which are not.

I can give you some examples from my own experience in which my own physicians or therapists have responded neutrally to my suggestions for such auxiliary help.

When I began to have problems with walking because the soles of my feet were tender, and my transverse arches had been flattened, a friend suggested that I get computer-designed insoles and special walking shoes from a firm in Seattle. I asked my doctor about the advisability of doing this. He was noncommittal, but wrote me an open prescription for orthopedic shoes that I was free to have filled anywhere I wished at my own expense. I did this, and have found the new shoes comfortable and helpful, although I find that it is necessary to wear them only on long walks, or shopping and other occasions when I will be on my feet for long periods.

I followed Karen Mahan's work with the computer-linked

biofeedback training in breathing control, so when she suggested that I use this as an aid in getting off drugs, I asked my doctor if he would recommend that. He said he had no objection, and told me to go ahead if I wanted to do so. He also checked my proposed withdrawal schedule and said it looked reasonable. I proceeded through the withdrawal without further consultation with him, and when I was through I reported my success to him. He said it was interesting, but apparently not interesting enough to ask me how I did it, or whether it might have any application for his other patients.

Likewise, when I was suffering from vasomotor rhinitis in the fall of 1985, I got a prescription for Seldane which successfully controlled the symptoms, but when the first prescription ran out, the symptoms came back somewhat as before. Karen had said she thought I could control the teary eyes and runny nose (and general malaise) with electromyograph and skin warming biofeedback methods. I borrowed some instruments from my daughter, and for about six weeks worked daily to bring up my skin temperature and relax the muscles of my face. By the end of that period, I was free of symptoms that have not come back during the following five years. I reported this to the ENT specialist I had seen, and he said, "Very interesting." Maybe so, but he was not curious as to how I had done it. *That* seems mighty curious to me!

It really does seem that doctors are not excited about hearing from patients who have been healed by someone other than themselves or by means they do not understand or control. While they can't deny these healings occur, they apparently don't have the time to extend their knowledge and expertise beyond the career tracks they are already on.

Let us look briefly at a few other modalities before winding up this chapter.

• **Hypnosis.** This is not exclusively a medical tool, but can also help patients to recall forgotten events or to perform necessary tasks from which they may consciously shrink. It does have legitimate medical uses, but these may be circumscribed by ethical considerations.

The difficulty I have heard expressed is that the hypnotist

may have purposes of his own that do not necessarily coincide with those of the patient. For example, the patient may want to regress to the memory of a specific event in order to illuminate subsequent behavior, but the hypnotist may be tempted to "show off" or exercise his own control by taking the patient on pathways that go beyond the original intent. I have spoken to two people who were successfully hypnotized, but who were disappointed by the results, because the hypnotist seemed to be using the exercise for his own purposes rather than theirs.

But if the hypnotist and patient agree on an appropriate goal, the suggestions received under hypnosis may help the patient to reach that goal.

• **Therapeutic massage.** Massage therapy, which is familiar to most people although they may not have tried it, is the best known of the touch therapies, but there are several others, all intended to promote relaxation, proper realignment of the muscles and other body members, better circulation of both the vascular and lymphatic systems, and enhanced digestion and elimination. There are connections to Eastern philosophies and techniques such as yoga and acupuncture, which are among methods used to free the flow of energies along the body's meridians. There are also schools of thought that teach that massaging various parts of the body, like the soles of the feet and specific pressure points on the hands, arms, legs, and ears are of benefit to particular organs—the heart, lungs, kidneys, and so on. There is no question but that these therapies and exercises do enhance relaxation, and most are benign so far as physical harm might be concerned. But anyone planning to receive whole body massage at frequent intervals might do well to clear such treatments with a physician, as massage that is too vigorous or too deep might be counterproductive with older people.

• **Acupuncture.** This modality is central to the practice of Chinese medicine, and in recent years it has become available in most parts of this country. It involves the stimulation of specific points on the body, usually by insertion of tiny, solid needles, which are then twirled. It is based on the principle that widely separated points on the body affect the functioning of certain organs, and these loci are connected along energy pathways called meridians. There are twelve such meridians on each side of the body, placed in symmetrical pairs. The purpose of acupuncture is to free the flow of vital energy along these pathways by stimulating the connected pressure points. Pain results when these flows are blocked, hence acupuncture not only relieves pain but can serve as an anesthetic in certain instances.

The acupuncture points may also be stimulated by using pressure, heat, cold, electricity, ultrasound, and even lasers to achieve therapeutic results. While many authorities consider acupuncture experimental, it has stood the test of time, and it is possible that more individuals have been treated by acupuncture in the course of human history than all other known systems of medicine combined.

• **Mentation.** This is a discipline known by that name only in my own city of Portland, where it was developed and practiced by Jim Samuels, the founder of the Mentat School. It uses a number of concepts and exercises well known in psychology, but not previously organized and systematized as Jim has done. It stresses the development of personal freedom and power, and enables its students to recognize how other people operate, and how to interface with them successfully and productively.

The critical area of mentation for most people is the "sorting" exercise. This enables the client, through structured sessions, to identify old stresses and relieve them, which lets the client keep his or her own emotional "garbage can" empty. The client is then able to accept new stresses until they, too, can be sorted and let go.

I have been through a good share of the contents of Jim's method, and have found it wholly pragmatic and workable as a personal psychological tool.

One of my interviews with Jim contained so much of his philosophy about healing that I believe it would be useful to include it here.

Doctors won't say illness is caused by stress, and they won't say it isn't. They are not adequately trained in stress-related disease. When you look at the person, you see an integrated system of mind, body, emotions, and self (and I would agree that 'self' and 'spirit' are the same thing). A physical symptom could easily be the result of an immediate cause from the body or any of the other three factors. I call my sorting exercise 'stress immunization.' Reducing a person's stress level can improve his health.

Doctors are beginning to accept that immunity involves more than the body—that is, that the immunity to stress is an index of self-esteem. It is the play between a person's vitality and his immune system. Sometimes all people need to get over disease is a change in environment to one that is more peaceful or pleasurable; stars, greenery, or whatever factors will make them feel more peaceful.

Age itself can be a stress factor. If we can make the mind and spirit younger, the composite age of the person will drop. The composite age is the sum of years registered on the body, on the mind, on the emotions, and on the spirit. A person can be ancient mentally and emotionally with a body age of thirty.

To remove stress, the first step is to find out where it is; that is, the locus of the incompetency in a person's experience, or inability to deal with life. The moment that is discovered, the person's competency begins to increase and relief of stress begins.

Another factor in stress is the double negative goal. This is a goal built on fear and resistance.

For instance, a spouse may resent criticism, and set the goal of avoiding criticism. On the face of it, this seems a wise decision, but it's a mistake.

The mind works in visualizations, or pictures. It will seek out whatever the individual concentrates on. The only way the spouse can successfully hold the idea of resisting or avoiding something is to picture it. So, while intending to avoid criticism, the mind actually concentrates more on criticism as if it were a goal. The result is increased sensitivity to criticism and stronger reactions to it as well. These reactions can make one sick.

The correct action would be to desire more support, validation, and compliments. When we concentrate on these, we feel better and begin the process of seeking them out. This is the road to recovery and health. The effort should always be to keep these goals positive.

Before we leave this brief review of healing modalities, we should consider the subject of placebos. A placebo is a medicine having no pharmacological effect, but is given to the patient who supposes it to be a medicine, as part of an experiment. It may also be given to a patient by a doctor in lieu of medication, but without telling the patient that it is a placebo. Ethical considerations aside, there are often cogent reasons for doing this.

In thousands of experiments and tests, it has been found that the number of subjects reporting relief from taking placebos, as compared to others in the tests given actual medication, runs consistently from 30 to 35 percent. This applies to all kinds of medicines and all varieties of symptoms and illnesses. The only rational conclusion is that those reporting benefits from taking placebos have believed that they were given the real medicine, and that they were going to get better, and they did. A corollary is that this belief, standing alone, is sufficient to make about one-third of all patients get better, regardless of medication or illness. Doctors giving "sugar pills" to patients in individual cases (not in tests) report similar success with patients who thought they were getting real pills. In many experiments, in fact, the placebos were at least as effective as the medications being tested, if not more so.

This being the case, one has to ask why doctors don't simply give up writing prescriptions, and give placebos to all their patients. The answer should be obvious. Even if this procedure resulted in one-third of all patients getting well, there would remain the sick two-thirds, who would still need real medicine to get help. Maybe they couldn't all be made better, but they certainly deserve the benefits of proven medications.

The point is really not whether patients should receive a given pill, but that the power of belief is so potent a force in healing that often no other treatment is required. The follow-on statement is that in caring for anyone, with any illness or condition, the basic ingredient in healing is the patient's belief in the

THE ART OF HEALING

efficacy of his or her own treatment.

Furthermore, if patients can be convinced of their own inherent power to heal themselves, in a surprising number of cases
they will be able to do so. It is important that they not be given
conflicting signals, and that the medicine or methodology can
be explained in a rational and truthful way. What this suggests
is that elderly patients be given medicines and other supports
that conform to their backgrounds and belief systems; otherwise
they may resist the treatment without quite knowing why.

An interesting example is found among the Indian tribes of
the American Southwest. White doctors working on reserva-
tions have discovered that the Indians have adapted quite well
to a system in which they go to the white men for medicines and
antiseptics for routine cuts, abrasions, infections, and so on, but
to their own tribal medicine men for mental, emotional, and
spiritual problems. I think this illustrates, in a pragmatic way,
the premise of this book.

# Part IV
# The Century of the Spirit

¶ *If the work you are doing isn't helping anybody
else, you are working for nothing in real terms.*

# 22. A Countess Through and Through

The Countess Stella Andrassy of Kingston, New Jersey, has done enough living, enjoyed enough creative successes, and suffered enough losses and physical pain to account for at least three normal lifetimes. Yet, at eighty-four years of age, she was still going full-bore on her inventions and cultural activities when I telephoned her in May 1991. The story of this remarkable woman deserves telling in some detail because of its inspiration in an age heavily infected by greed, self-interest, laziness, and defeatism. Who is she, and how did she achieve her present optimism and flair?

She was born to a wealthy Stockholm family and had a fine education. At five, she was a competent pianist. Early on, she'd learned the lesson of *noblesse oblige*—that if one is born to privilege, one does not deserve it unless one also shares it with others.

When she was a young woman, she met, fell in love with, and married a Hungarian count, Imre Andrassy, a military attache at his country's embassy in Stockholm. Later, she was swept up in her idyllic life in Hungary—a large estate, servants, private planes, and travel. They had three children, and Stella also found time to enjoy a succession of careers.

She continued her education in Budapest's academies. She

pursued her piano playing and the other rich cultural activities of the capital. She worked in a laboratory and helped develop a serum for leprosy. She published and edited an environmental magazine.

During the German occupation of World War II, the Andrassys were permitted to continue living at their estate, but when the Russian army pressed near in the spring of 1945, the couple fled with as many of their prized possessions as they could— paintings, antiques, an embroidered family seal, and relics of ancient civilizations. She recounted the story of their flight in *Pustam Brinner* (Swedish for "Prairie Aflame"), a book starkly describing that harrowing episode.

The Andrassys settled in the United States and pursued their scientific investigations, especially the uses of solar power, patenting some half-dozen devices.

But there were devastating losses during a single month in 1960. In that thirty-day period, Stella's grandson was killed in Vietnam, her brother and former nanny died, her arthritis flared painfully, and she lost her job. That period of loss and depression could have submerged her in a permanent funk. But out of it came another invention that has not only preserved her upbeat attitudes and lifestyle, but has given inspiration and hope to dozens of others. She calls it her Magic Circles. This is how she introduces her description of it:

Suddenly my secure world seemed to fall apart. The strokes of fate fell fast and hard. Within the brief span of three weeks, three of my most beloved ones died. At the same time, my health broke down, and I lost my job.

There I was, stranded in a foreign country, heartbroken, without money, and practically unable to walk. Stunned by the grim circumstances, I felt, most of the time, as if I were adrift in a tiny boat at high sea, surrounded by thick fog.

The long, sleepless nights were the worst, for then all my troubles arose to gigantic, ghost-like proportions that threatened to crush me. But in spite of my plight, I kept reflecting over how I possibly could lift myself up from the quagmire of self-pity and lethargy into which I seemed to be sinking.

If there was a way out, it evidently had to be something that did not cost money and could be done by somebody hobbling around on crutches.

Over and over again, I told myself: "You simply have to find a way to make your life worth living again."

Slowly, she says, a simple but workable plan began to crystallize. Its main features were these:

You must dedicate each day of the week to a meaningful purpose.

You must do something positive and productive every day, regardless of how small or insignificant the act may be.

These daily routines are repeated in the same order day after day, week after week, until, she says, they form a living chain. These are the seven elements of the Magic Circles:

*Monday* is dedicated to perseverance. Stella starts each Monday with a meditation period during which she affirms her strength and courage, and then prepares a detailed plan for the coming week. She makes a written list of activities, because "when I see my problems clearly written in black and white on paper, they somehow appear less awesome, and easier to cope with."

At the end of the week, she reviews what she has accomplished, giving herself a mental "pat on the back" for her successes, and resolving to keep her spirits up in spite of a few lapses. She then tears up the list and tosses it into the wastebasket!

"Through bitter experience," she writes, "I have learned that without tenacity and perseverance, no progress or improvement is possible. There are simply no free lunches. So I have printed on my pink lampshade my eleventh commandment: 'Thou shalt not stop trying!' "

*Tuesday* is the day for order. No longer enjoying the help of servants, Stella now does what is needed to keep her house in shape. She takes care of the disarray that needs attention most urgently, inside the house and in the garden. Her method is to deal with only one mess at a time, but when she tackles it, she does so wholeheartedly, working steadily and efficiently until it is done. Although her strength permits her to do this for only a few hours a week, she says it is amazing how it all comes together.

She also says it is essential to keep herself in tune with the spirit of what she is doing, because the petty chores would otherwise weigh her down. She reminds herself, "This is your home that you may clean! You are still capable of doing something—even if it is a lowly job. There is no menial work—only menial attitudes toward it."

*Wednesday* is the day of compassion in action. Compassion is more than a pretty sentiment, Stella says. It is *love in action.* It implies that you take part in, and identify yourself with, the suffering of others.

For her, this can be very painful, because with her inner eye she sees the suffering of starving children and desperate mothers in war-stricken countries. "All too well do I know what they are going through," she says, "because I was once one of them."

She admits it is hard for an ordinary person like herself to put compassion into action, but she does it in the simplest possible way. Each Wednesday she makes one phone call or writes one letter to a person who is lonely, sad, or sick. Also on Wednesdays, she tries to show a special kindness to someone, even to herself, to keep her mind, body, and spirit toned so she can maintain her work of compassion.

*Thursday* is the day of gratitude and remembrance. It's the day she meditates on her blessings. She recalls the beauty she has seen, the great music she has heard, the friendships she has made, and she thanks God for the love that has always been lavished on her by those close to her.

And as she has grown older, Stella is even able to be grateful for the difficulties she has gone through. For many years, she rebelled against the commandment "Bless those who persecute you and revile you," but now, strangely enough, she is able to do it. Not because they burned her home and killed many of her loved ones, but because they forced her to become strong and to conquer her fears. But she dwells mainly on happy memories.

She recalls the message of the sundial: "I count only the sunny hours."

*Friday* is the day of mind expansion. She believes that the elderly, more than others, need mental gymnastics to prevent their minds from going stale. On Friday evenings she does some serious reading, especially when she goes back to books which, like milestones, have marked the progress on her journey through life. Much of the information, and many of the ideas in these books, are associated with changes in her broadening perception of things. Other books are like refreshing oases in a barren land, helping her to renew her spirits as the week closes.

Most of the reading is directed, however. She makes notes as she reads, and returns to them the following week. The goal of her Friday reading is not only to acquire more knowledge, but also to gain deeper insight into things that really matter.

*Saturday* marks the accumulation of joy. She relaxes and takes it easy. She doesn't worry and doesn't hurry. Sad and disagreeable thoughts are banished.

When asked how she *creates* happiness, she replies, "Just look around. Look around, and listen; enjoy the sights and sounds and scents of creation.

"No day is so gray that you can't squeeze one drop of happiness out of it."

*Sunday* is the day of light—the most special time of the whole week. This is her chorus:

> Holy Spirit!
> Creator of Light and Song!
> Renew my strength,
> Augment my love,
> So I may better serve those
> Who need me most!

Later in the day, after a morning of meditation, she sits by a window where she can see the sky, and thinks about light in its many aspects. She visualizes the light present in all parts of the universe.

And she thinks about the inner light that has the power to

make her soul mature and unfold as fruit ripens and flowers bloom.

As the Sunday light fades to twilight, her mind comes slowly back to her body, and she hears a subconscious message: "Stop dreaming, put your feet on terra firma, and do your thing!"

So she prepares for another Monday spent in planning.

Stella Andrassy's brief essays on her Magic Circles have been put into booklet form, and she leaves a few blank pages at the end for others to use in adding their own ideas. She is willing to share this with any and all who communicate with her.

I have given this long report on Stella and her philosophy to make a most important point: There is nothing else on earth that duplicates exactly what Stella has done in her career, when she could have been languishing in a nursing home or sitting in a dark parlor with her hands folded in her lap, staring vacantly out the window. Through strength of will and a powerful creative drive, she has created this program, which works for her so splendidly, and could for others. In my view, this is the work of her spirit, of an inner spark for which mind and body alone cannot account. Most people her age have stronger, healthier bodies, and many have equally capable minds. But few can match that incandescent spirit that soars and soars, on wings that refuse to fold or break.

The purpose of this, the fourth and last section of my book, is to investigate the role played in human health by the spirit, and how the failure to appreciate this role is contributing mightily to the physical, social, and ethical ills of mankind. And as in the first three sections, I shall present my own perceptions and conclusions as to how these ills might be addressed and healed.

# 23. Diagram of the Whole Person

If Julius Caesar were writing this chapter, he would begin thus: *Omnes homines in tres partes divisi sunt—corpus, mens, et anima.*

Or, freely translated, "All human beings are divided into three parts—body, mind, and spirit."

This statement will be accepted by many readers at face value as common knowledge. But there may be some who cannot or will not do so because of their scientific or philosophical training. (It might be better accepted if Julius himself had actually written it.) These folks will likely say one of three things:

1. That the mind and spirit are the same thing, hence cannot be considered two different things.
2. That no physical evidence has ever been adduced demonstrating the existence of the spirit.
3. That there may be such a thing as the spirit, but it is not necessarily connected to mind and body, hence need not be considered in a discussion of health and human welfare.

To all these folk, I can say only one thing: "This is the end of the line for your present journey. If you cannot buy into this concept, even conditionally, please don't stumble as you get off the bus."

I think it would be unproductive for me to go into a philosophical argument to prove that the human spirit exists, as a separate entity, at this point. Thinkers and writers of many cultures have engaged in this pursuit for centuries, and are not much closer to agreement than when they started. But for all of them, and all of you, the recent news from the world's deepest thinkers in the realms of science and theology may be somewhat disquieting or reassuring, depending on your point of view. It is, briefly, that the quantum physics of recent decades has cut a good bit of ground from beneath the foundations laid by Newton, Descartes, and others, and cast into doubt traditional notions of reality, of certainty, and the immutable nature of the laws governing our physical universe. At the same time, theologists who have ventured into studies of time and space are finding less and less basis for ignoring the natural sciences in their constructs of deistic systems.

I use this figure of speech to illustrate my point:

Just as the two views on a stereopticon slide slowly merge into one three-dimensional picture as the two halves come into focus, so the divergent views of reality—the scientific and the theosophical—are bound to come into a stunning unity when more accurate views of reality are available to each side.

I'll go further into these developments in a later chapter, but for now, I'd like to deal with the nuts and bolts of our tripartite human structure, and show how all three must be integrated if we are to enjoy maximum and continuing good health.

The mind and spirit display such different aspects and functions that it will be useful to treat them as separate entities, even if they were to turn out not to be. The mind, for example, has the primary function of *thinking,* and for this purpose it commands that splendid biological computer, the human brain. In this activity the mind is largely value-neutral, running its programs through the brain in more or less objective and even-handed style and reporting its findings to the Person as a list of suitable findings or priorities.

The human Self, or personality, or character, however, is the spirit that has different and, if anything, more significant powers—those of volition, evaluation, intention, motivation, and, above all, *decision.* I offer this example that illustrates the distinction: When faced by a need for a difficult and harrowing decision, the mind is quite capable of making up lists of pros and cons, all the points in favor and points opposed, weighing on the problem in point. A neutral second party, looking at this list, might say, "There's no argument here—the answer is no, the guy shouldn't do it." But does that mean the guy involved is going to be equally logical, and come to the same conclusion? By no means—he is just as likely to do the illogical thing, especially if it involves the heavy emotions of relations with the opposite sex. His mind says "No," but his heart, or spirit, says, "Yes," and that's all there is to it.

In this activity, the spirit is supported and abetted by the will, certainly one of the least understood and most misrepresented components of the persona. The will, in my view, is one aspect of the spirit that a person needs in order to function at all, just as hands and feet are needed by the body.

Another aspect of the spirit is the conscience, which is similar, if not identical, to the Inner Guide described by some, the "still small voice" of many, and perhaps the governor or regulator by the technically inclined. The conscience might be considered just one component of the spirit if it were not that its unique performance suggests its connection to metaphysical sources outside the body. More on that, too, later on.

The mind/brain, whose interface is coming to light through studies in psychoneuroimmunology, is a tightly meshed servomechanism. It functions only as the spirit and will direct it to function, except that like all good machines, it is perfectly capable of idling along at any given speed, and of churning out all kinds of images and conclusions and speculations if it is not consciously directed to tackle a different problem. Exactly how the mind functions in this respect—that is, how it *thinks*—is a question that has never been fully answered, because it involves the interaction of physical and metaphysical forces. But the argument over how it works is guaranteed to keep our psychologists and philosophers busy through all seasons in both hemispheres, although modern man no longer thinks seriously in the summertime, when he is too busy getting a tan, playing golf, or fighting crab grass.

Thus we come to the body, which I think needs no further description or definition, except to say that it is often unappreciated by those who do not comprehend its miraculous construction and mystifying powers (which, of course, include the power of recovery from ills and the healing thereof).

This brings us to the emotions, often identified simply as "feelings." The emotions defy mechanical and statistical description, but play a critical role in precipitating action, stimulating or hindering decisions, coloring relationships, and otherwise having an impact on almost everything we think and do. I think the emotions are a curious blend of physical and immaterial forces, and cannot be assigned to any firm coordinates in the diagram of the whole person, or any sharply defined role in our thinking, or even any sure part in our spiritual lives. But they do exert a strong and often decisive influence in all three areas, sometimes simultaneously. We can see the devastating effects of this in some syndromes such as depression, which seems to have inputs and outputs from all segments of the personality.

At this point, I suggest that we undertake an interesting experiment. Let's open the 800-page volume, published in 1987 under the auspices of the American Medical Association, entitled *Family Medical Guide.* In seeking clues to various illnesses, and ways in which they should be treated, one would expect that a volume with this title and this many pages would cover all the important aspects of health and healing that an American family might need to know about. But what do we find?

Part I deals with the healthy body, and counts 65 pages.

Part II covers symptoms and self-diagnoses of illness, and includes 248 pages. There are more than 200 "symptom charts," of which 90 percent concern physical conditions and 10 percent mental or emotional conditions.

Part III describes diseases and other disorders and problems. It covers 485 pages, of which only 16 pages, or about 3 percent, concern non-physical conditions.

Part IV deals with the care of the sick. It has 32 pages, and is not subdivided into any categories of illness. Another 16 pages are devoted to accidents and emergencies, all of which deal with physical conditions or traumas. Interestingly, these do not include gunshot wounds (to self or others), knife wounds, or other wounds inflicted by assault, hence do not address physical trauma inflicted as the result of emotional upset or criminal activity.

So we see that in this entire volume, about 775 pages are devoted to physical ailments, their causes and cures, and only 41 pages to the mental or emotional—and no recognition at all that there may be such a thing as spiritual illness (more about this later). I think we can properly conclude that the American medical establishment is very strongly oriented toward dealing with the physical, to a very minor degree with the mental and emotional, and not at all with the spiritual.

From here we progress to the things that characterize the workings of all our parts. I think this will clarify many of the things I have been saying about the make-up of the human being.

First, I suggest that the entity known as the spirit also embraces the self, the character, the personality—all things that represent the essence or certain aspects of the spirit, but are not readily subsumed or made part of the concept of the "mind," as they often are. Yet, as "spirit," they must assert themselves as primary, or superior to mind and body, or the individual cannot function as an integrated construction. Direction and decision must come from the top, and this is the position of the spirit.

The characteristics of the spirit are both positive and negative, but all are decidedly discrete and not easily mistaken for something else. The positive aspects are such features as honor, courage, integrity, humility, modesty, determination, purity, and so on—often referred to as virtues. Negative traits are also readily identified, perhaps because they relate to factors usually referred to as evil or sin: lack of discipline or self-control, leading to excesses of greed, lust, or gluttony; laziness or sloth, leading to procrastination and non-achievement; pride, which destroys a person's acceptance by others, as well as his relationships; envy, the inevitable sidekick of pride; and finally anger, which promotes conflict and inhibits reconciliation. Deceitfulness is not often included in this list but it certainly belongs there, as it is reflected in lying, cheating, theft, and fraud. Taken together, the positive and negative aspects of the spirit comprise an impressive catalogue of personal attributes not easily confused with those of the mind or body.

The human will has its own set of characteristics, with the positive being such as decisiveness, perseverance, strength, and confidence; the negative are generally the mirror image of these.

Similar listings of the constituents of the mind, the emotions, and the body are so well known and exhaustively studied that there is little point in listing them here, except to note that many discourses in psychology may co-opt some of the characteristics I have assigned here to the spirit.

In the following chapter, I'll discuss a few examples of the working of the spirit in some of the everyday activities of human beings, to show that it is well accepted by the common man as being a distinct force in human affairs, and one that deserves all the credit it gets. That it is not so recognized by medical doctors for its overriding bearing on the health of people and society is a mystery I shall leave for others to solve.

# 24. The Ole School Spirit

I have to say, right up front, that the chapter you have just finished reading was one of the hardest of my career to write. I felt self-conscious, presumptuous, and a little naïve, for one good reason: I had almost nothing to guide me. Other writers have not met this issue head on—that is, describing, comparing, and locating all the elements that go to make up a human being. The reason, I believe, is that the scientists, wedded to the evidential, Cartesian model, simply don't include anything immaterial, much less spiritual, in their discussions. This includes the psychologists, who have wanted to get as close to the hard sciences as they can get, for many years past.

The religionists and spiritual writers, on the other hand, have been pretty much excluded from the field of practical philosophy by the scientists, who claim the cosmos as their turf and limit the discussion to the material, to that which is accessible to the senses. So the religionists have been limited to the inspirational or even the scriptural, which means there has been very little dialogue concerning what you might call natural theology, on the one hand, and an open, inquiring science that takes account of everything observable, by whatever means, even the human psyche or intuition.

So forgive me if I have sounded fatuous, uninformed, or kindergartenish. Believe me, I don't like it that way, but I have to write what I believe, regardless.

Now in the realm of everyday human affairs, we have the phenomenon of pervasive recognition of the role of the spirit in the least scholarly and philosophical of all fields, that of sports. Athletes, their coaches, and followers simply assume that without the proper character and spirit, teams don't have a chance against those better equipped in this regard.

Aside from the rah-rah or never-say-die spirit, and the "family" spirit of the greatest teams, athletes rely on their own spiritual strength in other ways. Take a look at this conclusion of a story in the *Portland Oregonian* for May 26, 1982, describing the recovery of Tony Conigliaro, a Boston Red Sox slugger, after being nearly killed when struck by a baseball.

> The doctors are not sure what brought about Conigliaro's partial recovery, and they are cautious about what lies ahead.
>
> One abstraction medical science will concede is the mystery of the human spirit, that of life which is neither bone nor tissue, but will. The same thing that enabled Conigliaro to hit a baseball after nearly dying from being hit in the head by one.
>
> "He's had experience in overcoming adversity already," his physician said, "and so, I suppose he's well prepared for yet another fight. I'm saying there is definitely a relationship between the fighting spirit of a person who is ill and his ability to survive an illness."
>
> The spirit soars, even as the body lies limp. The man who once roamed the outfields of major league baseball is climbing out of the valley of death.

Much better known, and the subject of a movie by the same name, is the Lou Gehrig story. It's hardly necessary to recount the conclusion of the story, when Gehrig stood in the infield of Yankee Stadium and bade his farewell to the choked-up crowd. More indicative of his indomitable spirit is his record of having played in 2,130 consecutive baseball games, despite bruising encounters with baseballs, fences, bases, and the bodies of other players; cracked ribs, chipped bones, broken fingers, broken toes, muscle tears, wrenched shoulders, pulled ligaments, and attacks of lumbago. That represented almost fourteen years of major league play without being out of the lineup, even for one day—a record that stands as the one least likely ever to be broken.

Well, you say, those examples are anecdotal, and can't be accepted as proof that the spirit has any role in human enterprise. In that case, my friends, I cannot convince you, because scientific proof is not possible, in terms of evidence in the scientific sense, because it can't be measured or quantified, or replicated in experiments.

But there is corroboration from many unrelated sources. Some of these, approaching the question from the scientific point of view, refer to the spirit as "consciousness," which I am willing to accept. However, I think that consciousness as such does not include the concepts of intention, volition, motivation, choice, or other factors such as values and morals that I hold are necessary to the human spirit for it to function effectively at all. But I welcome those people to the argument.

Dr. Fritjof Capra, author of *The Turning Point,* cited in Part III of this book, says this on page 296:

The nature of consciousness is a fundamental existential question that has fascinated men and women throughout the ages and has emerged as a topic of intensive discussion among experts from various disciplines, including psychologists, physicists, philosophers, neuroscientists, artists, and representatives of mystical traditions. These discussions have often been very stimulating but have also created considerable confusion, because the term 'consciousness' is being used in different senses by different people. It can mean subjective awareness, for example when conscious and unconscious activities are compared, but also self-awareness, which is the awareness of being aware. The term is also used by many in the sense of totality of mind, with its many conscious and unconscious levels. And the discussion is further complicated by the recent strong interest in Eastern 'psychologies' that have developed elaborate maps of the inner realm and use a dozen terms or more to describe its various aspects, all of them usually translated as 'mind' or 'consciousness.'

He then contrasts the Eastern and Western views of consciousness, pointing out that the Western or scientific view holds that it is a property of complex material patterns that emerge at a certain stage of biological evolution, while the Eastern view is a mystical one, based on the experience of reality in non-ordinary modes of awareness. These are achieved through meditation but may also occur spontaneously in the process of artistic creation and in various other contexts. Modern psychologists, he says, use the term "transpersonal" in describing this kind of perception, because it seems to allow the individual mind to make contact with collective and even cosmic mental patterns. His conclusion is that "we should therefore not expect science, at its present stage, to confirm or contradict the mystical view of consciousness."

On pages 359 and 360 of the same work, we find this paragraph quoted by Dr. Capra from Dr. Carl Jung's *Aion*:

Sooner or later, nuclear physics and the psychology of the unconscious will draw closer together as both of them, independently of one another and from opposite directions, push forward into transcendental territory—psyche cannot be totally different from matter, for how otherwise could it move matter? And matter cannot be alien to psyche, for how else could matter produce psyche? Psyche and matter exist in the same world, and each partakes of the other, otherwise any reciprocal action would be impossible. If research could only advance far enough, therefore, we should arrive at an ultimate agreement between physical and psychological concepts.

This, you will see, matches very closely my figure using the stereopticon pair, representing the scientific and metaphysical pictures of reality, taken from slightly different perspectives. We must understand that in the quotation above, Jung is using the word *psyche* to include both mind and spirit as I have described them, but his conclusion patently applies to both.

Some readers will detect an apparent discrepancy in what I have been saying. In one breath, I say that science and theology have been following separate, if sometimes parallel, paths—the science all material, the theology all mystical. In the next, I quote writers such as Dr. Capra who are talking about the convergence of the two, and about the increasing role assigned to "consciousness," which appears to embrace spirituality, in describing the total makeup of human beings. But the convergence, at least for the most part, including this case, is more apparent than real. This is because the admitted "consciousness" is still value-neutral, and does not embrace the very essence of spirituality and religion—the moral and ethical quality of existence, the need for some kind of standards if human culture is to advance in addition to surviving. I'll deal with this issue in later chapters, but I will say parenthetically that it is indeed *the* issue, if anything is to come of this kind of discourse.

A quotation from *The Little Book of Life and Death,* by D.E. Harding, is pertinent to this discussion. On page *vii* of his introduction he says, "Buddha cautioned that we do not take another person's word about existence, but rather experience it for ourselves."

Are we to take the word of a holy man about the very thing he is arguing? Only if we wish to give weight to the observations and experiences of his hundreds of millions of followers over a period of centuries. The point is that that long a period of testing by that many people is some kind of evidence of its validity. In medicine, they would call that an "epidemiological survey"—that is, drawing conclusions just by the sheer weight of numbers involved. If you think this is not a valid method, tell it to the American Cancer Society, which has just concluded a six-year study of the habits and lifestyles of two million Americans. I was one of the more than 100,000 surveyors used. If you can't determine anything from that, how are you going to do it?

It is necessary again to distinguish between spirituality and religion. The two terms are frequently and improperly used interchangeably. My dictionary defines religion as "a set of beliefs concerning the cause, nature, and purpose of the universe, especially when considered as the creation of a superhuman agency or agencies, usually involving devotional and ritual observances and often having a moral code for the conduct of human affairs." Subsidiary definitions suggest specific and institutionalized beliefs agreed upon by a number of persons or sects, and so on.

Spirituality, on the other hand, pertains to affairs of the spirit, which is the immaterial or incorporeal part of man in general, or an individual; or a supernatural, incorporeal being, as a ghost. This is the meat of it, although there are many corollary meanings growing out of that incorporeal aspect. Various religions have appropriated some aspects of the spirit into their belief systems and liturgies, but this does not alter the fact that the human spirit, in its universal manifestation, exists apart from any religious organization, and does not necessarily need to be identified with any particular religion, belief system, or manual of practice.

Many folks can be adherents of a religion throughout their lives, and never have a religious experience. Others can lead quiet, spiritually oriented lives without ever becoming associated with a religious group at all. A majority, perhaps, are involved in both areas, sliding in and out of spiritual perceptions while maintaining some kind of religious affiliation.

I'll break off this discussion right here, because I know that otherwise I'll surely become embroiled with one religious group or another, and I'll be at some degree of variance with at least ninety percent of them. I do believe that those who have developed their spiritual selves to a substantial measure will agree with much of what I am saying. Therefore, please don't search for any expression of creed or dogma, or support for any particular doctrine in these pages.

# 25. Spiritual Illness—What Is It?

In preparing to write this chapter I asked many persons, including priests and ministers, caregivers, and hospice house operators, how they respond to the question raised by this chapter heading. I also reviewed all the interviews, newspaper and magazine articles, and the books I have read on this subject. I found, somewhat to my surprise, that the phrase does not exist in common parlance.

How so? How can we be so devastatingly hung up on the illnesses of our minds and bodies, as we are, and still be oblivious to the health of our transcendent and (arguably) immortal souls?

This is a baffling question. I don't have an answer. But if any reader can prove I'm wrong about this, I'll gladly reward him or her with ten autographed copies of this book, plus a promise to reexamine the matter in the next printing.

It defies logic that we could be subject to all 99,999 physical ailments (including the relatively few mental diagnoses included in the five-digit code recognized by Medicare and by all participating doctors), yet not recognize that human health is strongly impacted by spiritual illness. If I told you that I think "character defects" and "poor self-discipline" are the same as this term spiritual illness implies, a few more of you might get on board. And there might be a few more when you learn that the renowned Carl Jung once said, "I have never met a person in the second half of life whose basic problem was *not* spiritual."

But we have to be aware that it is this kind of illness that is the earliest and most pervasive cause of the disintegration of the personality. People don't "fall apart" because they suffer from insomnia or fatigue, or simply because they have developed one or more neuroses or phobias; they are more likely to have these symptoms because of some weakness of spirit or character that has kept them from coping with life's demands.

What do I mean?

Consider a weakness such as laziness, a tendency often present from birth, which can destroy a person if not recognized and corrected early in life.

First of all, laziness leads to procrastination and that produces non-performance. We're always making excuses to ourselves: "I'll do that tomorrow—I don't have time right now. . . . I have to wait until I get my typewriter fixed. . . . That's just too *hard*. . . . I don't know where to begin. . . . They didn't tell me what format they wanted it in. . . . Maybe if someone would help me, I could do it. . . . I don't really understand what I'm supposed to do. . . . The other kids have already studied that, and I haven't, so what do you expect?. . . . I really need a break from all this, anyway. . . . I'll tackle it after I get all my stuff together, and get a little rest."

Sound familiar? It should, because it's one of the most widespread spiritual illnesses around. And under the name of sloth, it has made everybody's list of Seven Deadly Sins.

Or listen to this:

"I never get any breaks. . . . Joe got a pile of money when his father died, so he could get that car and take that vacation. . . . Lucy never had to worry about acne when she was in high school, so she was always popular. . . . Jeanie is so lucky—she can go to any store and buy a size 6 off the rack. . . . Phil just has a knack of getting along with people—they flock around him, but he's no smarter than me. . . . I wonder where the Evensons get their energy—they're going out almost every night, to shows or parties or something. . . . "

Sound familiar? Yes, another of the Seven Deadly Sins, called Envy.

Shall I go on? Shall I mention Pride, and Lust, and Greed, and Anger, and Gluttony? Is it too painful?

Yes, it's painful! Talk to any counselor, and he or she will tell you about clients who walk out after two or three sessions because they can't face the truth about themselves. The truth is too painful for anyone who lacks determination and courage to confront his or her weaknesses and do something about them.

Where is this leading? It is leading unavoidably to the need for *change*—personal, spiritual growth and *change*—if we are to do something about these pitiful, disintegrating lives of ours. If nothing is done, if the change doesn't occur before we enter our sunset years, the impact on our health and our lifestyles may well be devastating.

Dr. Scott Peck, in his fine book *The Road Less Traveled*, speaks constantly about spiritual growth, which he says, in effect, is the end of existence. He doesn't mention change *per se,* but without change there is no growth. The people who go to counselors and psychologists—if they are sincere—know in their hearts that they have to change if they are going to grow out of the messes and emotional traumas they have got themselves into. (They don't call this "spiritual illness," but they would have a clearer view of their problems if they did.)

Help for spiritual illness is hard to find. Those working with the mental aspects of it often have problems identifying it, much less knowing how to treat it. Psychiatrists, as we have said earlier, are trained to diagnose and treat their patients' mental illnesses. My own hunch is that they fail to spot many of the things I have described as spiritual illness, for one of two reasons: Either they haven't been trained to look for it, hence cannot make the causal connection with the patient's symptoms; or the patient, being human, is too experienced in hiding his or her own fatal flaw.

Dr. Peck describes a woman client whom he couldn't help for a long period because he hadn't been able to make a diagnosis. (He is a psychiatrist.) Other kinds of counselors for mental problems do not attempt to diagnose these ills directly, but believe that only the clients themselves can do this if they are led along the right path—and can be persuaded to keep their

THE CENTURY OF THE SPIRIT

feet to the fire until they discover what their core problems are. People will dodge and weave and avoid the simple truths about themselves, but find they recover rapidly when they do face the facts and "bite the bullet."

As I wrote in Part II in discussing the New Medicine Man, ministers of the various religions are often poorly situated to provide the right kind of counsel. For one thing, they don't have much training for it. For another, they may lack the personality, the skill, or the desire to become proficient. For a third, they simply don't have time, because spiritual healing is very time-consuming, and there are dozens of more immediate demands on their agenda. And for a fourth, many ministers themselves are "burning out" and inwardly screaming for help.

An article by Hank Whittemore in the April 14, 1991, issue of *Parade* magazine was entitled "Ministers Under Stress," with the subhead, "More and more members of the clergy are feeling overwhelmed by the demands of their ministries." (Reprinted with permission from *Parade,* copyright ©1991.) He cites the testimony of Roy Oswald, a senior consultant at the Alban Institute, a non-denominational organization based in Washington, D.C., that offers consultation, leadership, training, and referral services for churches and synagogues nationwide. Oswald estimated that seventeen percent of the parish clergy he has worked with in more than twenty years of consulting are suffering from long-term stress or burnout. He says many of these wounded healers are reaching out for help through counseling and psychotherapy—or "hitting bottom" before winding up at professional treatment centers around the country.

Such stress includes the expectable factors such as alcoholism, drug abuse, overeating, or other addiction, not to mention "carnaling out," or becoming sexually involved with parishioners.

One such pastor resigned his pulpit because, he said, he was gradually being worn down by subconsciously becoming trapped by the "walk on water" syndrome—the notion that, "because you're a preacher, you can accomplish anything. . . . I did not have a crisis of faith, but of emotion and energy. It's almost impossible for leaders of a congregation to accept that their pastor needs pastoring. So I began to strangle on my anger, finding myself unable to sleep and even losing interest in studies I love. . ."

He's now "out of the system" and counseling other ministers who confidentially seek his advice.

The problem of spiritual illness has a poignant significance for the elderly as they approach life's end. A great many of them, perhaps a majority, have suffered some kind of character defect or "missing bricks" in their personality structure during their lifetime, but have plastered these over by making lots of money, "buying off" their family members and friends with entertainment and gifts, by moving to a new locale every so often, by travel or constant activity—but these can no longer compensate for their hidden lacks after the money runs out, or a supporting spouse dies, or they become disabled (physically, mentally, or emotionally) to the point that these substitutes can no longer be enjoyed. Then, with some kind of unguessable accounting staring them in the face, they find they are approaching the final passage through the dark door at express-train speed. They "drug out," they claw at their loved ones for some kind of support, they drive their doctors crazy with their continual complaints. "Maybe tomorrow I'll find out what's wrong with me," they say.

Deep inside, they know darned well what's wrong. They've waited too long to make their peace with their fellow human beings and with their God, and now they want someone else to help them through that final rough passage.

Yet others achieve peace of mind much earlier in life. One wire service story reports that about half of all elderly people die peacefully and without pain. The obvious difference is that the latter "did their laundry" when they still had time.

In his *Road Less Traveled*, Dr. Peck also picks up the theme that people face the need to endure the hardships they encounter, saying, "the attempt to avoid legitimate suffering lies at the root of all emotional illness." This is close to what Dr. Gerald Jampolsky said about fear and addiction in Part III of this book— that fear drives people to separate themselves from God and from each other, and to compensate by reaching for pills, alcohol, cigarettes, chocolates, and so on. This is a perfect prescrip-

THE CENTURY OF THE SPIRIT

tion for the final fear that strikes as death approaches, when it's too late to make the changes that could have been made twenty or thirty or forty years earlier.

Dr. Peck reinforces this point, and echoes my earlier statement, by saying that most of his patients avoid lofty goals and hard work: ". . . they are content to be or ordinary men and women and do not strive to be God."

So how many people *do* strive to be God? In most contexts, this reference to "God" is simply a metaphor for "being the best"—that is, winning an Olympic gold medal, becoming president of the United States; in other words, shooting for the top. The fact is, you will never hit a target higher than your aim. If you aim low, to be a second-level manager, you will be lucky to get that high. If you aim higher, you may not get the top job, but you will never know if you don't try.

There are many applications of this principle. Napoleon said: "Every corporal carries a marshal's baton in his knapsack." He knew; he had been a corporal himself, and became Emperor of France, higher than all his marshals.

I had a friend who was a vice president of a large bank when he suffered a heart attack. Later, he calmed down and had a long and pleasant career, retiring as vice president. He told me, "After I realized I was never going to be president, things got better and I have felt fine ever since." His ambition almost killed him, but the question now is: Could he have been happy if he had never aspired to the top spot? In his case, the answer almost certainly is "No."

I've known many young men who, in their late twenties and thirties, became very active in civic organizations and enterprises, and who mistook their early success and public approbation for a sure route to the top in business. But the first doesn't translate into the second. A large degree of experience and seasoning is necessary before the head of a large business will help a young buck to ascend to the top echelons (unless, of course, he is the president's son). But I know of no case in which Junior First Citizen survived all the pitfalls of notoriety—arrogance, adulation, the dancing attendance of sweet young things, and their junior peers—to become a senior first citizen. It takes unusual self-knowledge and discipline to know when to modify goals that were too lofty for the individual concerned to begin with. But my first statement holds: You'll never know if you don't try, and you won't make it if you don't shoot for it. Just be realistic and be wise enough to shift your aim when the odds become too great.

Dr. Capra's book *The Turning Point* is useful once again in considering the role of personality (in my terms, read "spirit") in illness. On page 328 he writes:

It is becoming apparent that the patient's personality is a crucial element in the generation of many illnesses. Prolonged stress somehow seems to be channeled through a particular personality configuration to give rise to a specific disorder. The most convincing link between personality and illness has been found for heart disease, and links are being tentatively established for other major diseases, notably cancer. These results are extremely significant because as soon as the patient's personality enters into the clinical picture, the illness becomes inseparably linked to his entire psyche, which suggests the unification of physical and psychological therapies.

Exactly! Dr. Capra might object that he has said nothing about spirit here, but if you divorce spirit from religion, I think you would agree that there is no good reason not to make this substitution, because we are talking about the same thing (i.e., spirit = personality). I have already discussed this, and I will accept the terms *psyche* and *character* if we include the spiritual dimension, which includes an orientation to values and judgments.

Dr. Capra continued by saying that "the psychosomatic nature of illness implies the possibility of psychosomatic self-healing. The first step in this kind of self-healing will be the patients' recognition that they have participated consciously or unconsciously in the origin and development of their illness, and hence will be able to participate in the healing process. In practice, this notion of patient participation, which implies the notion of patient responsibility, is extremely problematic and is vigorously denied by most patients . . . associating the idea with blame and moral judgment."

I realize the force of this when I look back at an illness of my own in late 1980, when I almost welcomed a diagnosis of cardiac insufficiency as justifying my weakness and irregular heartbeat. When I was given an angiogram to check the condition of my cardiac arteries, I was secretly hoping for a finding that would require open heart surgery, which would prove that I had not been kidding about the way I felt.

But I didn't get it. The arteries were clear. And from there I went on to my eventual passage through biofeedback and mentation therapy, and the series of realizations that enabled me, seven years later, to get rid of my medications entirely. I no longer take prescription medications of any kind except for an occasional antibiotic or antihistamine. Yes, I'm somewhat arthritic, but I don't take pain pills. Yes, I have occasional stomach or intestinal upsets, but I don't take antacids. Yes, I often feel a cold coming on, but I don't take cold pills. I get bed rest and stay warm and concentrate on feeling good, which I have my doctor's permission to do. I avoid rich food, liquor, or coffee after 6 P.M. (and not much before!) and spend at least eight hours in bed every night, come what may. Why get sick?

Dr. Capra does deviate a bit from the standards I set for myself when he says that the notion of personal responsibility must be limited and relative, and "like free will cannot be associated with absolute moral values." This is a strange statement, and smacks of the relativism that is causing so much havoc in other areas of life. You see, this can be a cop-out that lets everybody off the hook. How can you be *partly* responsible for something? Where, on a scale of 0 to 100, should we stop? If I said, "somewhere between 40 and 60," most people would probably agree. But in application, you'd find most people willing to accept a responsibility factor no higher than 10 percent, and very few would fail to object to a number higher than 90.

It is tempting to explore the concept of spiritual illness further, because the mind is full of images that beg for elaboration. But in the interest of time and space, not to mention the reader's concentration span, let us see why spiritual health is vital to the mental and physical health of the individual, and perhaps to the community and nation as well.

# 26. Integration—What and Why

We have been leading up to the theme of this chapter—the integration of the body, mind, and spirit to achieve total health. The Romans said, *"Mens sana in corpore sano"* (a sound mind in a sound body). If one segment is ailing—or even a segment of a segment—the whole is ailing to some degree.

Perhaps we should begin our inquiry by quoting Wilma Mankiller, the principal chief of the Cherokee Nation. Addressing a gathering to study health care for minorities in Portland recently, she said that mainstream medicine has always ignored traditional tribal medicine, which has a history spanning thousands of years.

Mankiller received life-threatening injuries in a traffic accident and consulted with tribal healers concerning some aspects of her situation. She said the tribal medicine gave her the mental and spiritual strength necessary to undergo a kidney transplant.

American Indians have always had a holistic approach to health and medicine, and their healers—the medicine men—are trained in psychic and spiritual healing procedures as well as physical aspects of medicine. Concerning the latter, many Indians now seek the services of Western doctors for their admittedly advanced techniques of diagnosis, surgery, and medication, but rely on their own medicine men for other kinds of healing.

I ask this question: If proper methods of diet, rest, and exercise are needed for physical healing, are there not counterparts that people can use for their mental and spiritual health? Of course there are.

This is very apparent in the case of the mind. The mental diet should indeed be "food for thought." We should be at least as careful of what we put into our minds as we are with food for our bodies. We need a balance of good reading—informative, broadening non-fiction; magazines and newspapers to keep up with events and trends; the electronic media, TV and radio, for up-to-the-minute periodic reports, as well as entertainment and visual input; a spice of humor and satire, and even a certain amount of heavy stuff, the heaviest we can digest—science and religion as in this book, for example (if you have made it this far, you have enough heavy stuff for this year, at the least). That's the way to give our minds the nutriment they need to live and grow on.

Mental rest is important, something few people think about. If we keep our minds in a whirl all the time, we're going to wind up tense and edgy even though we have not stirred from our chairs. Perhaps ironically, physical exercise is often the best way to rest our minds. The calm and relaxation we enjoy during a long walk through the woods can be a wonderful mental—even a spiritual—restorative.

When you're taking a "couch break," and certainly in bed at night, learn how to take charge of your thought processes, and do not allow yourself to be caught up too often in daydreaming that is too stimulating, exciting, or demanding (on the positive side), or too worrisome, scary, or depressing, on the negative side. How do you do this? There's no set rule except practice, but the basic principle is, instead, to focus on something pleasant and positive—memories of childhood, planning for a vacation, or working out details of some project you are about to undertake. This latter has always been good for me—just thinking through how I am going to set the tiles in that closet, how the plywood should be handled around a projection, and so on. If you just want to let your mind idle, put it to work on lists of names or places you want to remember. There's no end result here, and if you're interested in sleep, your list-making can merge at any time with slumber.

Some of this comes under the heading of mental exercise, except that there's no result expected from nap-time thinking. But if you don't do this while lying down, give your mind a workout some other way. Many experts in the field of gerontology say flatly, "Your mind is a tool—use it or lose it!"

Sometimes there's a lot of wisdom in the letters and comments that appear in the advice columns in the newspapers. You just have to be smart enough to tell the wisdom from the other stuff. In a recent "Dear Abby" column in the *Oregonian*, I saw this challenging headline: YOU'LL NEVER LIVE TO BE 90 BY THINKING YOU'LL DIE AT 70. There followed a letter from a correspondent past 90, who submitted a positive version of the humorous list of things that tell us when we're growing older, such as "you sit in a rocking chair and can't get it going. . . . Your knees buckle but your belt won't," etc.

He headed his column, "You Can Stay Young When . . ." and followed with, "You quit dreading old age and realize that life begins at retirement; it's your second chance at life—your opportunity to do all the things you've always wanted to do but never had the time; you will know you are staying young when you stop thinking you're getting senile because you forgot something that wasn't important in the first place," and concludes:

> Our Creator gave us brains so we can make our own decisions. Then he gave us a choice of living 70 or 100 years, so you need not join the 68 percent who were healthy enough to reach 60, but never made it past 75 (their own mental attitudes set the dates of their funerals).
>
> The 32 percent who are staying young are positive thinkers who like it here and are determined to stay as long as they feel useful and needed. It's a great world—why leave it? [Taken from the "Dear Abby" column by Abigail van Buren, copyright ©1990. Reprinted with permission of Universal Press Syndicate. All rights reserved.]

An article in the February 1991 issue of *Longevity* magazine described how six famous people keep their minds active and lucid in their later years. This is how they do it:

Glynis Johns, 67, actress and ballerina, treats her brain like a muscle. She assumes it will atrophy if she doesn't use it. "When I'm not learning lines for a part," she says, "I still commit something to memory, such as passages from the Bible. If I don't keep up the memorizing process between roles, it takes me much longer to learn my lines when I'm working."

Actress Estelle Parsons, 64: "I remember hearing years ago about an English repertory actor who learned a new piece of Shakespeare every day to keep his mind fresh. I keep mine honed on poetry. I also memorize a lot of things just because I want to know them."

Walter Matthau, actor, 70: "I read a lot, listen to music, which I find mentally stimulating, and walk about five miles a day and observe people and things. I still think of myself as 21."

Oscar-winning actor José Ferrer, 79: "I keep my brain cells stimulated with music (mainly classical and jazz) and by reading books in several languages—English, Spanish, French, and Italian. I have an insatiable curiosity and wish I could live to be 300 to learn more."

Trial lawyer Melvin Belli, 83: "If you retire, you stagnate and lose all the vibrancy and vitality that lawyers who go to court every day have. So I still practice law and oversee a twenty-lawyer firm that handles about a thousand cases per year."

Dr. Norman Vincent Peale, 92, minister, lecturer and author of *The Power of Positive Thinking* and other books: "I believe that everything you've stored in your subconscious is there for instant recall when it's needed. If you work with your subconscious, it tries to serve you; if it doesn't, it's because it hasn't been trained. Practice asking it for information daily. The mind doesn't grow old and tired unless you let it."

Another article in *Longevity*, this one appearing in the March 1990 issue, was headed "Anti-Brain Aging." After citing considerable research into the physiology of cell loss and other factors in Parkinsonism and Alzheimer's disease, it concluded thus:

Some of the most intriguing evidence that an active brain stays young into advanced old age comes from the laboratory of Marian Diamond, Ph.D., of the University of California at Berkeley. Diamond has found that rats who are stimulated by what she calls 'toys'—swings, ladders, wheels, treadmills—develop bigger brains than their cage mates and maintain brain function longer. Even if they are only spectators, watching younger, more frolicsome animals at play, their brains benefit. On an average, they are still alert and curious at three years of age—the human equivalent of 90 years.

This evidence . . . suggests that 'exercising' the mind keeps it fit and youthful, just as physical exercise keeps the body in shape. As for humans, Diamond says, "If you don't use it, you lose it."

But one person can't tell another what the right exercise is for him or her. I think there should be an element of recreation in it—doing it for fun as well as for benefit. If you've tried different things and don't enjoy them, or have trouble staying with them, try something else! The variety is infinite. Here are just a few I jotted down in a couple of minutes:

- Reading of all kinds (the more you vary it, the better).
- Taking night school, community college, or graduate courses.
- Tutoring students, or adults needing language and math skills.
- Counseling others through SCORE (Service Corps of Retired Executives) and other programs.
- Serving on citizens' advisory committees, or in public life.
- Leading youth groups.
- Dramatic, music, and dance groups.
- Elderhostel, Great Decisions, etc.
- Working on political campaigns, including initiative or referendum drives.
- Trying out new recipes and sharing them with friends.
- Taking day trips to places of interest you have not seen before.
- Exchanging letters with a pen pal in another country.
- Working with a high school or college alumni group.

And the list goes on.

When it comes to spiritual health, the problem is much more than avoiding spiritual illness—even if you have succeeded in getting all that cleaned up. Many if not most people have never experienced really robust spiritual health, at least since early childhood, and this is always true of those who have allowed themselves to be trapped by negative patterns of thinking and feeling. They may not know how it *feels* to enjoy spiritual integrity, for example, assuming that they could define it, or recognize it if it were to appear.

This is not the place for a homily on cleaning up your act, but I discussed it in the chapter on spiritual illness. My perception is that spiritual health, or wholeness, is the same thing as spiritual integrity—that is, that there are no cracks or seams or holes in the character; weaknesses that threaten to make it impossible for a person to do and say the right things at all times, and to go to sleep with a clear conscience every night.

This is difficult only if you have made no effort over your lifetime to work toward integrity, to practice it, and to eliminate those characteristics that inhibit it. The formula is really very simple (even though the practice is hard). It is set forth in this verse from the Bible: "All that is required of you is that you do justly, think rightly, and walk humbly with your God."

That's *all?* That's *all!* And that is a lot—it's everything!

There are many excellent books on the market that suggest ways of doing this, but two of the best I've seen (listed in the bibliography at the end of this book, along with many others) are:

*Minding the Body, Mending the Mind,* by Dr. Joan Borysenko, a Bantam New Age book, published by arrangement with Addison-Wesley Publishing Company, Reading, Mass.

*Notes on How to Live in the World, and Still Be Happy,* by Hugh Prather, Doubleday and Company, Garden City, N.Y.

Dr. Capra, who has been quoted several times previously in this book, is helpful on the subject of integration also. On page 234 of *The Turning Point,* he writes:

"Indeed, our experience of feeling healthy involves the feeling of physical, psychological and spiritual integrity, a sense of *balance* among the various components of the organism and between the organism and its environment. This sense of integrity and balance has been lost in our culture."

My response to this last sentence: Regarding a sense of integrity and balance having been lost by an entire culture, he can be right only in a broad sense; in individual cases, yes and no. There are certainly many who enjoy this sense of wholeness, and just as certainly, many more who do not.

But note that, as I suggested earlier, Dr. Capra describes integrity only as a feeling or sense of wholeness. It is not, by itself, a specific characteristic like the virtues and vices I have described. Thus it is always a composite of many other things, and has no existence apart from its constituents. But we are painfully aware when it is lacking.

Note that we are aware when we lack that integrity; that we can work to achieve or restore it by repairing or resupplying its constituents; and that we know it has reappeared by the way we feel when we can calmly inspect our inner selves, by meditation.

I hope this whole chapter has not come across as a "holier than thou" sermon. That's the risk you run when you discuss morality and ethics—people will think you claim to possess the virtues you describe. But I have to work as hard as the next guy to achieve anything in this realm, and I know by sad experience that you can't achieve static perfection—you have to work at it all over again every day. You can slip into that good feeling of being integrated for a few moments and then slip right out again. "Eternal vigilance is the price of peace"—and so it is of integrity also.

# 27. Morality, Ethics, and Responsibility

The nation was shocked recently by the results of a survey that was described in the 270-page book *The Day America Told the Truth—What People Really Believe about Everything That Really Matters*. The book was written by James Patterson, chairman of J. Walter Thompson, one of the world's largest international advertising agencies, and Peter Kim, director of Research Services and Consumer Behavior for the same firm. Based on questionnaires filled out by 5,700 people at fifty locations across the United States, the survey produced a portrait of a nation without a common morality.

"Americans are making up their own rules and laws," the book concluded. "We choose which laws of God we believe. There is absolutely no moral consensus in this country as there was in the 1950s and 1960s."

Among the findings, according to news reports announcing the book's release, were these:

- Only 13 percent still believe in all of the Ten Commandments.
- Nine out of ten citizens lie regularly.
- Nearly a third of all married Americans have had an affair.

❦ A fifth of the nation's children have lost their virginity by age thirteen.

❦ One in seven Americans carries a handgun, either with them or in their cars.

❦ One in five women says she has been date-raped.

❦ Seven percent of Americans would kill a stranger for $10 million.

The release of the book's findings produced a flood of responses, some echoing distress at the state of the nation's morals, others expressing skepticism concerning the validity or interpretation of the survey, or the significance of its findings if true. I'm not going to get into that. But I think the survey, more clearly than anything else I have seen, reinforces the point I made in an earlier chapter—that there is such a thing as spiritual illness, and that it is rampant among large segments of our population.

A critical factor that will not escape most thinking people is the close connection between some of these findings and the wave of philosophical relativism that seems to have engulfed a lot of us in its suffocating sophistry. We hear it expressed in terms such as these:

"Of course there's such a thing as obscenity, but it's a relative matter. If it's a true reflection of life, and doesn't do any tangible harm to anybody, it's probably okay."

"I have a right to take a few pencils and envelopes home from the office once in a while. I sure put in enough overtime that I never get paid for."

"You can't expect people to work at top speed eight hours a day, even if they do get coffee breaks. They should just work at a speed that's comfortable for them, and not have to meet quotas just because somebody else thinks they're reasonable."

"Of course I took a couple of days off to go skiing when I was at that conference in Colorado. The fact that I had my expenses paid had nothing to do with it—I went to the conference, didn't I?"

I think most readers will see the relativism in these statements, but perhaps it is most obvious in the last. We'd probably get a unanimous vote that one day of skiing after a five-day conference is justifiable, and certainly not grounds for discipline. The same panel would also vote unanimously against the propriety of five days of skiing after a one-day conference, at the sponsor's expense, unless it was specifically authorized.

So where do we draw the line? It's a relative matter, isn't it? And is it surprising that human beings usually make these decisions in their own favor, and against the interests of the sponsors or employers?

But take the really shocking statement that seven percent of survey respondents would kill a stranger for $10 million. That is relativism at its absolute worst. The commandment says, "Thou shalt not kill" . . . period. What are we to gather from this? That an even larger percentage of respondents would kill for $100 million, or $1 billion? Or that a smaller number would do it for $5 million, or $50,000? Do you see what I mean by relativism— that is, it depends?

I'm reminded of the guy who sent the IRS a check for $25, with this note: "Dear IRS: I underpaid my income tax last spring, and I haven't been sleeping well since then, so I'm sending you a $25 check. If I find that I still can't sleep, I'll send you the rest."

Another excellent example is found in the parable of the rich young man who sought to become a follower of Jesus. The latter told the young man he would be welcome as a follower—all he had to do was to give up all his possessions and join Christ in his ministry. Immediately the questions arose: "*All* my possessions? What about my house? *All* my clothing? *All* my gold and silver, for which I worked so hard? *All* my horses and sheep and cattle? *All* my servants? That's asking a lot!"

The answer, of course, is *all*—yes, *all.* This is very difficult for people to understand, because on the face of it, it seems so unfair. Yet the young man had to make that choice if he was to take up his new vocation. Just a parable? Not really—it speaks to our time also. It speaks to the requirement for commitment if we are really to undertake a new career, a new direction. At work, in marriage, in the organizations we join, we can't expect to come in part way and be successful. We can't have part of our mind saying, "I'll sneak some time off now and then so I can keep doing a little selling on the side." We can't try to keep an old flame alive while we're trying to build a life with a new one. We can't run a trade show for the sponsor and still take commissions from an exhibitor to get him a good location and publicity. But it happens all the time!

The principle I want to espouse, and want you to accept, is that there are indeed absolutes in the realm of morality and ethics, and individuals do not have the license to compromise them. There is no difference between a man's integrity in his public life and in his private life, although some well-known politicians would like to have us believe that there is. It is immoral to cheat, even a little bit; it is immoral to lie; it is immoral to plagiarize the work of another, even one sentence or idea, without giving credit; it is immoral to fudge on the measure we give for a measure received; it is immoral to be a day late on a project we pledged to complete at a time certain (do I hear howls of protest?); it is immoral to provide favors for one person or class, if promised for all; it is immoral to retain for ourselves what is intended for others as well; it is immoral to keep the extra change if the clerk makes a mistake at a restaurant or store; it is immoral to falsify records, reports, references, endorsements, financial statements, or any other paper or document upon which others rely as reflecting our true knowledge or opinion; all these things, and hundreds more, are immoral, and offensive to right-thinking people. But how many of us are accustomed to fudge, fudge, fudge from the moment we awake in the morning until we go to bed at night? No wonder we have a hard time sleeping!

I've had problems of this nature, large and small, all my life. I have had a tendency to take on more projects than I could handle. Then I make excuses for being late or for doing a less-than-adequate job. We know when we are not giving 100 percent, and it bothers us—or certainly should. Eventually, we either learn, and reform our ways, or we take the other road and go on doing whatever we can get away with. Very likely we'll wind up cheating ourselves by indulging in booze, dope, gambling, or other excesses. We're not hurting anybody but ourselves, you say? Well, I think that's immoral too, because when you hurt yourself you are going to hurt other people as well.

So what are the standards? If there are absolutes, how are we to know them?

There are many answers to this question. Businesses and organizations, and virtually all governmental bodies, have codes of ethics that are variously based and just as variously enforced. Religious organizations offer guideposts and sets of rules. Wise friends, doctors, lawyers, teachers, psychologists, and others can provide good advice. If we are observant and intelligent, we can also, to some degree, learn from experience. This calls to mind a well-known saying: Good judgment comes from experience, and experience comes from bad judgment. The force of this saying is that if you don't want to learn from the experience of others, you're going to have to go through the bad-judgment period yourself, because nobody is born with good judgment.

The real answer, the final answer, however, rests not with others but with ourselves. Our own standards should be higher than any we find in the marketplace, because no compromise should be involved in ours. It's dangerous to think, "It's okay for me to do that, because our code of ethics doesn't forbid it." How many times do you hear public figures defend themselves by saying, "I haven't done anything illegal"? That may be a legal defense, but it isn't an ethical defense. A better attitude would be, "Our code of ethics says it's okay, but I'm not going to do it, because it just doesn't feel right."

In the end, it comes down to a matter of integrity, of single-ness of character and purpose, of giving the same answer no matter what the circumstances, insofar as the rightness of an action is concerned. It comes down to being the same person, making the same decisions, whether you are in your own living room at home, in a hotel room in Las Vegas, on the first tee at Pebble Beach, on a non-stop flight to Tahiti, dickering with a rug merchant in a Moroccan bazaar, or debating philosophy with an Oriental bonze. Let's not get into an argument about observing cultural niceties or "going with the flow" in a sticky situation; we're not talking about things that are truly relative such as prices and negotiable obligations. We're talking about bedrock character, about keeping your word, about not deceiving others, about avoiding temptation, even though it might make you unpopular to do so. In other words, about integrity.

When I have run into an argument on this issue, it is not so much about the desirability and need for a return to moral values; it is about where the responsibility lies for teaching these values to those who follow us. Some say, "The parents must do this at home." Some say it is a job for the schools, because kids are hearing too many different things in their home environments. Still others say the teaching of morals and ethics should be left to the churches, because these are religious issues, and tax-supported agencies shouldn't get involved.

I say it's an issue for all three of those, for society as a whole, and certainly for every human being as an individual. If moral responsibility is taught at the mother's knee, and then at school, and then by youth groups and educational directors, and then in job training programs and then in business and industry, people will get the idea that nobody is going to act as their consciences, and they'd better get their act together before they're halfway through their twenties.

I hardly have to give you examples. Too many young athletes, some with multi-million dollar contracts in their jackets, have destroyed themselves with dope and booze before they have had time to prove themselves on the field. Too many young actors and celebrities have done the same thing, often adding a variety of pills to the fuel that sends them spinning out of control. There's something terribly wrenching about seeing this beautiful young person, so arrogant and feeling so omnipotent today, lying on a cold marble slab in some morgue tomorrow, all because of the lack of inner control.

Well, I can't get so wound up that I get away from the theme of this book. But this discussion leads me to a critical point that I have expressed in other ways in other places—that all the ills that grow out of character weaknesses, whether these ills show up as physical, mental, or spiritual disorders, remain and must be dealt with in old age if not earlier in one's life. Past indiscretions, old lies, old enmities, old regrets, old sins of omission and commission, old slurs and slights, old failures, old psychic and emotional traumas, are still there, but even more powerful because they have become all tangled up with each other, and because there is now less energy and fewer handles with which to control them. Besides, there are fewer offsetting joys and diversions, and much less time remaining to deal with them.

Am I too preachy? I am not concerned; I'm speaking the truth. Let him hear who will listen. I'm not the first person who has said these words. Three thousand years ago, King Solomon told his subjects, in the first chapter of Proverbs, "Wisdom cries aloud in the open air, she raises her voice in public places; she calls at the top of the busy street and proclaims at the open gates of the city: 'Simple fools, how long will you be content with your simplicity?' "

So there's no secret or mystery about any of this. It's just that so few people seem to want to do the hard work of thinking and doing what they should be thinking and doing. On all sides we hear, "I could never understand algebra . . . it's too hard! I can't write a decent sentence; all that grammar is too hard. . . . I could never learn Latin . . . it's too hard. . . . I couldn't learn to knit like that, or lay bricks like that, or build a fence like that . . . it's too hard!"

Too hard . . . too hard . . . too hard! That's all we hear. But then we see people from all stations in life who don't believe any of that, and who just go ahead and do it, without any fuss or complaint.

Then we hear that society has a responsibility to see that everyone has three square meals every day, and a roof over his or her head, and medical care, and a decent job, and an education, and someone to look after Junior while Dad and Mom are at work, and freedom from want, and freedom from fear . . . yet who's going to do the hard work needed to pay for all those goodies? Well, you know the answer better than I . . . the other guy, of course! It's easy for you, and it's easy for the guy in the next block, but it's just too hard for me!

From the fury of the Norsemen, and the tyranny of the tax collectors, and the whining of the "too hard" crowd, dear Lord, deliver us!

# 28. Evolution and Spiritual Growth

Voices are now being heard throughout the civilized world, suggesting that a historic turning point is at hand. It heralds the pending merger between science and theology, a merger that will follow the 300-year schism that has separated the two like the Berlin Wall. I have mentioned and defined this schism in earlier chapters, pointing out the persistent influence of earlier thinkers such as Descartes and Newton, barring intangible evidence from scientific inquiry. This is a subject on which I should not express an inexpert lay opinion, but will quote from several sources.

Edgar D. Mitchell, an Apollo 14 astronaut, expressed the unity principle very clearly: "There are no unnatural or supernatural phenomena—only very large gaps in our knowledge of what is natural."

In the same vein are the words of John Polkinghorne, chaplain of Trinity Hall, Cambridge, and a former professor of mathematical physics at Cambridge University. In his book *Science and Creation* he writes:

> One of the most powerful human motivations is the need we feel to make sense of our experience, to gain a coherent and satisfying understanding of the world in which we live. It is a quest which unites science and theology in comradely concern, for they are both attempting to explore aspects of the way things are.

He distinguishes between the kind of theology identified above, and the theology propounded by religious figures, by using the term "natural theology," which he describes thus:

"Natural theology may be defined as the search for knowledge of God by the exercise of reason and the inspection of the world."

Many religionists dispute the validity of this concept, holding (in the words of Karl Barth) that God cannot be known by the power of human knowledge, but is apprehensible and apprehended solely because of His own freedom, decision, and action.

It is neither necessary nor possible to resolve this historical philosophical dispute here. If we accept the concept of natural theology, however, we shall more readily understand how and why scientists are willing to engage in discourse with its proponents as they have found few points of engagement with the more dogmatic or esoteric religionists.

To quote further from Polkinghorne:

Those imbued with thirst for understanding will not find that science alone will quench it. . . . That the world is intelligible is surely a non-trivial fact about it and the basic laws and circumstances of the universe exhibit a delicate balance which seems necessary if its processes are to evolve such complex and interesting systems as you and me. It is surely inevitable to inquire if these facts are capable of a more profound comprehension than simply the statement that they are the case. If that further understanding is to be had it will be beyond the power of science to provide it.

After many more pages of discourse, Polkinghorne concludes by writing:

We have come to the end of our discussion. In its course, science and theology have encountered each other in a way that seems, to me at least, to be characterized by fruitful interaction rather than mutual friction. Einstein once said, "Religion without science is blind. Science without religion is lame." His instinct that they need each other was right, though I would not describe their separate shortcomings in quite the terms he chose. Rather, I would say, "Religion without science is confined; it fails to be completely open to reality. Science without religion is incomplete; it fails to attain the deepest possible understanding." The remarkable insights that science affords us into the intelligible workings of the world cry out for an explanation more profound than that which it itself can provide. Religion, if it is to take seriously its claim that the world is the creation of God, must be humble enough to learn from science what the world is actually like. The dialogue between them can only be mutually enriching. The scientists will find in theology a unifying principle more fundamental than the grandest unified field theory. The theologian will encounter in science's account of the pattern and structure of the physical world a reality which calls forth his admiration and wonder.

Polkinghorne has set the stage in an attractive and encouraging way, but he does not address any proofs other than the perceptions of a scholar steeped in both the mathematical and religious traditions. It is hard to challenge his position because he has not given us any substantial theorems to challenge.

Thomas Berry, in his beautiful book *The Dream of the Earth*, has one entire chapter in which he discusses the unfolding changes in relationships between science and religion. Entitled "The New Story," this chapter holds that the traditional roles of the two philosophies have been antagonistic, but that this has to be modified in both cases in light of developments that have rendered them progressively unrealistic. The impasse of the redemptive Christian community, he says, is that it has grown apart from history and from the earth story as well. The impasse of the secular scientific community is the commitment to the realm of the physical to the exclusion of the spiritual. But he says there is a remedy: to establish a deeper understanding of the spiritual dynamics of the universe through our own empirical insight into the mysteries of its functioning.

"In this late twentieth century," he writes, "this can now be done with a clarity never before available to us. Empirical inquiry into the universe reveals that from its beginning in the galactic system to its earthly expression in human consciousness the universe carries within itself a psychic-spiritual as well as a physical-material dimension. Otherwise human consciousness emerges out of nowhere."

Dr. Fritjof Capra, in *The Tao of Physics*, devotes the entire volume to exploring the consonances between modern quantum theory and the philosophies of the ancient Chinese and Hindu sages. This view is well expressed by J. Robert Oppenheimer, as quoted by Dr. Capra:

> The general notions about human understanding . . . which are illustrated by discoveries in atomic physics are not in the nature of things wholly unfamiliar, wholly unheard of, or new. Even in our own culture they have a history, and in Buddhist and Hindu thought, a more considerable and central place. What we shall find is an exemplification, an encouragement, and a refinement of old wisdom.

The limitations of pure science are considered by Dr. Capra in these words:

> The realm of rational knowledge is, of course, the realm of science which measures and quantifies, classifies and analyzes. The limitations of any knowledge obtained by these methods have become increasingly apparent in modern science, and in particular in modern physics which has taught us, in the words of Werner Heisenberg, "that every word or concept, clear as it may seem to be, has only a limited range of applicability."

Many residents of the Western nations are yet unaware of the great degree to which traditional notions of matter and motion have been made obsolete, at least in part, by quantum mechanics and the implications of Einstein's theory of relativity. The deceptively simple equation $E = mc^2$ tells us straight out that energy (E) and mass (m) are not only convertible into each other, but that this conversion takes place at a uniform rate in proportion to the square of the speed of light.

That's just plain hard to grasp intellectually, for anybody. This story is told: A few years after Einstein had proposed his revolutionary theory, one young scientist was discussing it with a renowned older scholar at a meeting of savants. The younger man remarked that he had heard that only two people in the world, besides Einstein, understood the theory. Responded the older scientist, "I wonder who that other man might be!"

But the theory has been substantiated in many ways since it was pronounced. Witness atomic fission and fusion, for example. In fission, enriched uranium is bombarded by neutrons, released when there is enough material in the pile to reach a critical mass. In the process, the uranium breaks down into two other substances which, together, have slightly less mass than the uranium itself. This loss of mass is compensated for by the release of huge amounts of energy, in accord with the Einstein formula. In the process of fusion, on the other hand, hydrogen is converted into helium at the rate of four hydrogen atoms to one of helium—all very tidy, according to the periodic table of elements, except that the mass of the helium atom is slightly less than that of the four hydrogen atoms. Result: a corresponding release of energy, a process that makes the N-bomb a bomb, and not just an interesting piece of hardware.

Werner Heisenberg, early in this century, contributed the uncertainty principle, which holds that certain pairs of attributes of particles, such as their position and velocity, cannot be predicted with complete accuracy. Position alone, yes; velocity alone, yes; but the two together—no.

There is also the wave-particle principle, which states that under some conditions, small amounts of matter behave as particles, while under other conditions, they behave as waves. It becomes very difficult for a layman, educated in conventional physics, to understand that sunlight consists of waves, in terms of frequencies, but alternatively of particles, described as photons, because of the characteristics of mass they exhibit, such as pressure. Is sunburn caused by the oscillation of the waves or by the impact of the particles, causing the skin to heat, or both? A layman's question, and the layman (myself) doesn't know the answer.

The net effect of all these discoveries has been to make scientists much less cocksure about the universal, unchanging aspects of some of its laws, while, at the same time, giving religionists a different slant on the way "creation" works. One thing upon which modern thinkers and writers agree is that the entire universe, all its matter and energy, all of its forms of crystal, light, and life, are interconnected in one way or another. This has made human beings considerably more reluctant to engage in activities that materially change the environment, because it is impossible to predict where the chain of cause and effect will lead, and what the end results will be.

A fitting conclusion to this phase of our discussion is found in the recent book *A Brief History of Time* by the British scientist Stephen Hawking, who points out that the current dichotomy between science and religion has the scientists describing *what* the universe is, while the philosophers are too busy catching up to ask *why*. Hawking says that any complete theory explaining the origin and destination of the universe should be understandable to anyone, not just to a few philosophers and scientists. He then concludes:

> Then we shall all, philosophers, scientists, and just ordinary people, be able to take part in the discussion of the question of why it is that we and the universe exist. If we find the answer to that, it would be the ultimate triumph of human reason—for then we would know the mind of God.

What does all this have to do with the problem of health care for seniors? I think it doesn't require a great leap of imagination to see that if the most profound thinkers of our time are viewing the problems of science and religion in the same light, and governed by the same sets of rules, it doesn't make sense to keep the practice of medicine, on the one hand, completely walled off from the ministrations of religion or spiritual counselors, on the other. Just as the two disciplines are approaching a common focus on a universal level, so medicine and spirituality should join their resources to combat ill health of all patients, and seniors first and in particular because of their pressing spiritual needs.

I have gone to some length to present the scientific progress of recent years to emphasize another point, and that is that modern conventional medicine is still pretty much stuck in the Descartes-Newton mode of experimental evidence, which requires attention only to those things accessible to the five senses, and to nothing immaterial. In view of the fact that perhaps seventy-five to eighty percent of all adult human ailments are attributable to non-mechanical or non-material causes, this makes the current emphasis on mechanical and material remedies all the more questionable.

But even more important than the issue of illness and healing, in my opinion, is the issue of right behavior and the responsibility of people not only for the present welfare of society, but more important, for the direction taken by humanity in the future. The history of evolution shows us that its very essence is dynamism; humanity, and other life forms, are never static. The very clear message is that humans of our generation, as of every preceding generation, are even now determining what forms and directions humanity will take in the near and distant future. I am totally opposed to the "Brave New World" model of selective breeding to determine our future direction, just as I am opposed to any state-directed efforts of any kind to make that determination. This does not mean, however, that we cannot make intelligent choices that will lead to a richer cultural matrix in which our young will grow, and an improved moral atmosphere for the development of ideas and institutions that stimulate and shelter growth.

I propose specifically that a book covering these very issues, or a scholarly anthology based on the questions and comments posed in its pages, be made the basis for study in at least one course in the humanities in high schools and colleges throughout the United States. That's something our young people could get their teeth into; and it shouldn't create any problems that could not be resolved by presenting the options put forward by the various schools of thought. It's the stuff of controversy, of intellectual ferment, and it would be the best thing in the world for students of all ages to sharpen their teeth and whet their intellectual knives on.

Dr. Peck, in *The Road Less Traveled,* states unequivocally, "Believing that the growth of the human spirit is the end of human existence, I am obviously dedicated to the notion of human progress." Farther along, he says, "Discipline . . . is the means of human evolution," and follows by saying that there is a force, or motivation, lying behind discipline, and that this force is love. He defines love thus: "The will to extend one's self for the purpose of nurturing one's own or another's spiritual growth." I had a hard time appreciating the meaning of this, until I realized that growth implies *change,* and that the ability to change one's self and the course of one's life lies behind all improvement and all progress. In my experience, people can change, and do change, and have the power to change themselves in the direction they want to go. Thus the question is not just spiritual growth, but what *kind* of growth, and what *quality* of growth. I think that for a person to decide to change, and actually to change, is an act that is divine in nature because of its very creativeness.

In contemplating this question of growth, we experience another realization. It is that the process of being "born again" is not simply the peculiar belief of a particular religion; it is a profound truth of deeply spiritual psychology. It implies the total release from all that existed yesterday in the form of misconceptions, prejudices, prerogatives, fears, animosities, jealousies, rigidities, inhibitions, anxieties, and so on, to become completely open to new information, new slants on old problems, fresh starts, and new relationships. (The new relationships are not necessarily with new people, but may be simply new relationships with old friends, relatives, and family members.)

By becoming truly new people we become clear of old offenses in our own minds and in the eyes of God. We gain new understanding of the injunction: "Except ye come as a little child, ye shall in no wise enter the kingdom of God." And by becoming clear, and open, and innocent, we likewise stand at the very threshold of a state of grace, awaiting only a nod from the infinite to enter therein. There is no other feeling in the universe that can match that feeling.

It is not impossible to live so as to be reborn every morning, and thus to greet each day with pure joy and thankfulness. I refer doubters to the story of Stella Andrassy with which I opened this section.

This process, however, does not free us from commitments and responsibilities. I see a vast dilemma confronting us, and society in general: If we control our own evolution, toward what shall we choose to evolve? There are many models, perhaps scores or hundreds, but I can suggest two. One is based on traditional American individualism, which sees strong people making the most of their opportunities, and carrying themselves as far as they can go in their chosen directions. The second is the group model, the cooperative one, with society moving more or less in concert, and people conferring and helping each other to surge ahead in slow but unrelenting waves.

It seems to me that these two models, which we might term individual and collective, sort themselves inevitably into male/female terms, the male being the strong, often lonely, single striver, and the female being the nurturing, supporting, unifying group adherent. This conforms perfectly to the Chinese formulation of yin and yang. There is a real question whether society as a whole can evolve in both directions at once, in terms of a pronounced advantage either way, or whether some compromise, or tightly-woven, compound model may be available. I wish only to suggest that when we set our personal goals, we keep very much in mind what will happen to society (meaning, first of all, our families and friends and communities) if we succeed in reaching them.

I should also point out that evolution is not necessarily toward favorable growth or desirable goals. The story of the rocks is full of evidence of races of living things that have been too successful for their times, and have grown fat and lazy during times of sunshine and plenty, only to lose their capacity, if not their will, to adapt and to survive. The lushest, prettiest plants are not those most likely to come through a long, hot summer. So remember that growth per se, or success at the feed trough, does not always mean survival into the next geological age.

If I have been successful in thoroughly confusing my readers concerning psychology, philosophy, religion, science, creation, and evolution, it has been in large part deliberate. The worlds of science and religion are scenes of great argumentation and confusion when their dons and experts gather in earnest conference. Few "laws" and dogmas are held sacrosanct any more, as the quest for objective reality and the place of life and consciousness in the cosmos becomes more urgent and more frenetic. I invite the reader to continue his search for information by checking out some of the books in my bibliography, by paying attention to the wealth of information in the media, and pursuing lines of inquiry according to his or her own tastes. It's a fascinating quest, and the near future holds new wonders for nearly all those below the age of ninety. Good traveling!

# 29. Looking Ahead

We're near the end of the line, where the bus stops, and we all have to get out and continue by ourselves. This is an excellent place in our deliberations to do this, because our look at the evolutionary process in the last chapter is a natural lead-in to my next perception.

Not too long ago I read a book entitled *A New Science of Life* by Dr. Rupert Sheldrake. The main thing I got out of the book was the author's suggestion that before evolutionary changes can occur, perhaps a modified template or model needs to be designed by whatever intelligence is responsible for the creation of the universe—but that once it has been designed, it then becomes possible for prototypes fashioned by this template to come into existence anywhere in the world, or perhaps even in the universe.

Without going into the author's rather esoteric arguments and examples, this suggests to me that perhaps the idea of the New Medicine Man is such a template. There are models and templates of a very similar nature struggling to appear in many places, as outlined in Parts I and II of this book, simply because of the great vacuum that exists in the gap between conventional medicine and the softer, or mentally and spiritually oriented modalities. I think it is just possible that the formulation I have presented may represent the creation of a template for a definitive form of operator who can take that role, and assume that title, and fill that void.

Not surprisingly, doing all this research and writing has stimulated my own thinking, and led me to conclude that I would be a pretty sorry type if I did not get involved in some such activity myself. I currently have a proposal in process to provide free consultation to a large health organization interested in the possibility of developing a staff of senior peer counselors, and we'll see what comes of that. I'm probably not the best prepared or most highly qualified candidate around, but I'm sincerely interested in seeing exactly how this might prove out in practice.

One thing I intend to be insistent upon, and recommend that anyone else so inclined insist upon the same thing, is that senior volunteers in this field provide an overall "plus" service to their suffering fellow elders, and not simply step into the shoes of paid staff who continue to occupy their offices and draw their salaries, while leaving most of their former duties to the volunteers. This is never the overt intention of the staffers concerned, but can easily be the practical result if all parties are not aware of lines of responsibility, and the nature and amount of the real work being done.

A special problem exists in the case of elderly members of minorities in the very large metropolitan areas, whose needs are easily overlooked, and who are not practiced in the art of getting attention and support. It's fairly easy for senior peer counselors to work in their own communities, with elders of the same economic and cultural backgrounds, but another matter to get something started in the slums and ghettos that, sadly, exist in every large urban center. I don't really have a formula for this, but I'm aware that quite a few people are active in this area, and I could only hope that some would see the need for New Medicine Men with some expertise in dealing with the less fortunate whose needs might be even more overwhelming.

We must again look at the economic storms that loom ahead for health care of all kinds, and be aware that if we are realistic, we shall be less dependent on public resources of all kinds—especially financial—and more inclined to look at private and volunteer support for effectuation. In the private sector, there are always other resources, in manpower and in kind; but in the public sector, there is seldom any "other." It is always money, or paid manpower, or both, but beyond that, not much. This suggests that any discussion or planning should not become too tightly bound to plans that depend on funding for implementation, while leaving wide scope for any interested parties—individual, organizational, or corporate—to get on board.

I have to say that, in my observation, most of the true healing in this country is being done by women. Nurses of all degrees and backgrounds play a huge role. They do a large share of the communicating done in doctors' offices with older patients who need explanation, reassurance, reminding, a friendly touch, and an ear to listen to their multiple fears and frustrations.

At all the conferences and workshops I have attended, where attendees have been from all parts of the country, women have been in a large majority. They have an instinct for what is needed and to relate readily to many of the suggestions I have made, because this conforms to their work experience. They also seem to be less self-oriented and defensive of their own positions. One of the statements I have heard frequently is, "This might have worked but we got involved in a turf battle."

Therefore, if there is to be a shift of models away from conventional medicine toward a broader-based system depending at least partly on alternative methodologies, I think we must be prepared for much less shift of financial and organizational resources than of people and programs involved. The establishment will pretty much keep what it already has, in terms of government recognition, financial support, and organizational structure. The people moving away from these structures, along with volunteers attracted to the cause, will have to make do with no more resources, but accept other forms of compensation.

I think most of those committed to the healing arts will agree that the greatest compensation for their work is love: first the love of those they have helped, and then the love of God for helping Him in His work. If one's work isn't helping someone else, one is working for nothing in real terms.

There are a few comments I want to make, and I haven't found another good place for them, so I'd better get them off my chest here.

The well-maintained human body is like the wonderful one-horse shay. The parts all function perfectly for years and years— 90 to 100 years in most cases—until it just wears out all at once, and collapses in the middle of the road, as it were. But the spirit isn't like that at all, and that's what makes its care and nurture so important. There is no reason why the human spirit should not continue to grow throughout life, and become stronger until one dies. Each time a spiritual illness is overcome, each time one gets rid of an undesirable trait or habit, each time a new realization bolsters confidence or increases understanding, the spirit is expanded and strengthened. This is different from everything in the material world, which, no matter how many times it is straightened or smoothed, always tends to fold or crack in the same old place. Sure, you can add splints and bindings, and weld more patches over the surface, but the basic stuff of matter can't be "healed" in the way the human spirit can. So take care of what you have, and help it grow!

I had planned to devote a chapter to communication with the non-material entities in the universe, but concluded it would contribute little to this discourse. I do suggest, however, that the one way you can do the most for yourself is to learn to meditate in an open, sincere, humble, and persistent way. There are different means of doing this, and many good essays or little manuals on how it is done. Find one that suits your background and tastes, and just do it. You will get out of it exactly what you put into it, and the rewards can be great.

There may be questions about the soundness of many of my ideas and suggestions. I have had to cover so much ground that I haven't even tried to do a work of thorough scholarship, which would have required a far greater amount of reading and research than I have had time and energy for. But if you will look over the list of people who have helped me and given interviews (at the end of this book) I think you'll understand the scope of their interests and expertise; and the fact is that I have received support and validation at almost every point. Virtually to a person, they have told me, "You're singing my song! Go to it! Someone needs to be saying this!" So encouraged, I've plodded ahead, although admittedly I've received suggestions for enough additional interviews that I could have doubled the number actually done. Without the support and validation I have received, this book would never have gotten off the ground.

The most striking example of this occurred in Allentown, Pennsylvania, during a trip I made in November 1990, to cut a tape for a syndicated TV program. Between my hotel and the restaurant where I had breakfast, I passed an office building with a glass door on which I read, "Lehigh County Area Agency on Aging." On the last morning, I passed the building after 9 A.M., when the offices were open, and decided to go in.

Cold turkey, I approached the receptionist, and after a deal of explaining, succeeded in getting her to summon a case worker. This turned out to be a pleasant woman named Joan Schnalzer, who said she was on emergency duty; but when I explained where I was from, and the kind of information I was developing for this book, she said, "Come on in. I guess you're an emergency."

She told me feelingly about the needs of older people from all levels and lifestyles in her county, and the urgency of providing services to them. The last thing she told me before I left was, "You realize I couldn't have done this by myself. My personal and spiritual beliefs are one reason for my interest in helping and working with people." Her eyes were moist as I left, and I thought to myself, "The story is the same here as it is in Portland and Seattle, and surely the same in California, Maine, and Florida."

So I have left my heart hanging out in the open by publishing this book—my heart, that mysterious organ that represents the whole human being better than anything else. It is of the body, the very stuff of existence, that can stop the whole enterprise just by ceasing to beat; it is also the symbol of love, which is just the spirit in action. And the heart is linked so closely to the brain and mind through its network of nerves and emotions that we cannot separate the functions of any single component. When we say we are thinking with our hearts, everyone knows exactly what we mean. And when people say, "Ya gotta have heart," we agree that without the courage and perseverance of that organ, no enterprise can succeed against opposition.

From the beginning of this work, I have known that I had to do it, and that I had guidance and outside help from other than human sources. I certainly could not have done it on my own. The same force was at work during my twenty-four years on medication, and my ultimate withdrawal from it. I couldn't have done that alone, either. I have had three mottoes that have kept this support in the forefront of my mind:

The first: Sufficient unto the day is the strength thereof (just to get through the next twenty-four hours).

The second: Put on therefore the armor of God, and no man shall prevail against you (when fears arose from the risks I took in speaking and writing in the public forum).

The third: I can do all things through Christ which strengtheneth me (when I felt doubts as to whether I was capable of doing a hard thing). This is the phrase Dr. Norman Vincent Peale gives the losers who have come to him for advice and spiritual strength.

I'll give you two more that my father used to heal himself, without medical supervision, when he had some type of heart problem at age sixty-seven: "Go to the ant, thou sluggard," and "Take up they bed and walk." This was just pure affirmation and visualization, and it worked until his death at age eighty-three in an automobile accident.

In my meditating over a period of time, I became aware that my thinking and attitudes become clearer if I hold a few positive key words in mind whenever I want to position myself in relation to any circumstances that arise. If I stay within a little cube at the center of things, with eight words at the corners of the cube, everything else will come right. The first four words, representing abstract reality, are Truth, Beauty, Joy, and Freedom; the other four words, representing concrete, personal reality, are Light, Life, Love, and God. You need no clothing or protection from any winds that blow if you just stay inside that cube.

This is my own Zone of Interior, the strong base from which my expeditions are launched. This is not dogma or doctrine; simply my own experience and truth. Others may use different words and different ways of accessing their own spiritual support, but it may help to know it is there. If you are sincere and persistent and wholehearted, you will find it.

It is this perception, which seems to be finding an echo in many other venues of philosophical, religious, and ethical and moral thought, that leads one to conclude that the twenty-first century will likely see a marked tide toward reincorporating spiritual values, activities, and influences into our lives. That is why I titled this part "The Century of the Spirit."

THE
END

# Bibliography

Aitken, Robert: *The Mind of Clover.* San Francisco, North Point Press, 1984.

Bailey, Covert: *Fit or Fat.* Boston, Houghton Mifflin, 1978.

Berry, Thomas: *The Dream of the Earth.* San Francisco, Sierra Club Books, 1988.

Borysenko, Dr. Joan: *Minding the Body, Mending the Mind.* New York, Bantam Books, 1988.

Brown, Dr. Barbara: *New Mind, New Body.* New York, Bantam Books, 1975.

Burns, Dr. David D.: *Feeling Good: The New Mood Therapy.* New York, William Morrow and Company, 1980.

Burrows, Ruth: *Fire upon the Earth.* Denville, N.J., Dimension Books, 1981.

Capra, Dr. Fritjof: *The Tao of Physics.* New York, Bantam Books, 1977.

——— *The Turning Point.* New York, Simon & Schuster, 1982.

Cohen, Gene D.: *The Brain in Human Aging.* New York, Springer Publishing Company, 1988.

Cousins, Norman: *Anatomy of an Illness.* New York, Bantam Books, 1981.

——— *Human Options.* New York, W.W. Norton Company, 1981.

Dawkins, Richard: *The Blind Watchmaker.* New York, W.W. Norton Company, 1987.

Feldenkreis, Dr. Moshe: *The Elusive Obvious.* Cupertino, California, Meta Publications, 1981.

Fensterheim, Dr. Herbert: *Stop Running Scared.* New York, Dell Publishing Co., 1977.

Fisher, Dr. Donald: *I Know You Hurt But There's Nothing to Bandage.* Portland, Touchstone Press, 1979.

Freudenberger, Dr. Herbert J.: *Burn Out.* New York, Bantam Books, 1980.

Fried, Dr. Robert: *The Hyperventilation Syndrome.* Baltimore, Johns Hopkins University Press, 1987.

Greenlick, Dr. Merwyn R.: *Health Care Research in an HMO.* Baltimore, Johns Hopkins University Press, 1988.

Graedon, Joe & Teresa: *50 + —The Graedons' People's Pharmacy for Older Adults.* New York, Bantam Books, 1988.

Harris, Dr. Thomas: *I'm OK, You're OK.* New York, Harper & Row, 1969.

Hastings, Dr. Arthur C. et al: *Health for the Whole Person.* New York, Bantam Books, 1981.

Hawking, Dr. Stephen: *A Brief History of Time.* New York, Bantam Books, 1988.

Jacobson, Dr. E.: *Progressive Relaxation,* Second Edition. Chicago, Chicago Press, 1938.

Jampolsky, Dr. Gerald: *Teach Only Love.* New York, Bantam Books, 1983.

Justice, Dr. Blair: *Who Gets Sick?* Los Angeles, Jeremy Tarcher, 1987.

Kushner, Dr. Harold: *When Bad Things Happen to Good People.* New York, Shocken, 1981; Avon, 1983.

Landry, David: *Culture, Disease and Healing.* New York, Macmillan, 1977.

Lewis, C.S.: *Surprised by Joy.* New York, Harcourt Brace Jovanovich, 1955.

Maltz, Dr. Maxwell: *Psycho-cybernetics.* New York, Simon & Schuster, 1969.

Norfolk, Donald: *Executive Stress.* New York, Warner Books, 1989.

Peale, Dr. Norman Vincent: *The Power of Positive Thinking.* Englewood Cliffs, N.J., Prentice Hall, 1961.

Peck, Dr. M. Scott: *The Road Less Traveled.* New York, Simon & Schuster, 1978.

\_\_\_\_ *People of the Lie.* New York, Touchstone Books, 1985.

Pelletier, Dr. Kenneth: *Mind as Healer, Mind as Slayer.* New York, Delacorte Press, 1977; Delta, 1978.

Polkinghorne, John: *Science and Creation.* Shambala Publications, Boston, 1988.

Prather, Hugh: *Notes on How to Live in the World and Still Be Happy.* Garden City, New York, Doubleday, 1986.

Progoff, Dr. Ira: *Process Meditation.* New York, Dialog House, 1980.

Rosenbaum, Dr. Edward: *A Taste of My Own Medicine.* New York, Random House, 1988.

Sanford, John A.: *Dreams and Healing.* New York, Paulist Press, 1978.

Saward, Dr. Ernest: *A Tale of Two Cities.* Lecture, one of series sponsored by Kaiser Permanente Center for Health Research, Portland, 1989.

Sheldrake, Dr. Rupert: *A New Science of Life.* Los Angeles, Jeremy Tarcher, 1981.

Siegel, Dr. Bernie: *Love, Medicine and Miracles.* New York, Harper and Row, 1988.

——— *Peace, Love and Healing.* New York, Harper and Row, 1990.

Simonson, Dr. William: *Medication and the Elderly.* Rockville, Maryland, Aspen Systems Corp., 1984.

Simonton, Dr. O. Carl: *Getting Well Again.* Los Angeles, Jeremy Tarcher, 1981.

Stearns, Ann Kaiser: *Living through Personal Crisis.* Chicago, Thomas Moore Press, 1984.

Wing, R.L. *The Illustrated I Ching.* Garden City, New York, Doubleday, 1982.

Wolfe, Dr. Sidney and staff: *Worst Pills, Best Pills.* Washington, D.C., Public Interest Research Group, 1988.

# List of Collaborators and Interviewees

Adams, Joseph, retired assistant dean and director of public relations, Oregon Health Sciences University.

Bauman, Ivo, retired chairman, Mt. Angel Telephone Company, Mt. Angel, Oregon.

Bogardus, David, pharmacist, McCann's Pharmacy, King City, Oregon.

Buell, Joan, former director, Hospice House, Portland.

Colling, Joyce, Ph.D., gerontologist, Community Services Department, Oregon Health Sciences University, Portland.

Deale, Alan, DD, pastor, First Unitarian Church, Portland.

Dunlop, Jean, RN, MA, staff supervisor, Alcohol and Chemical Dependency Program for Older Adults, St. Vincent Hospital, Portland.

Durham, Mary, Ph.D., assistant director of research, Group Health Cooperative of Puget Sound, Seattle.

Eskeli, Christopher, Ph.D., director, Alcohol and Chemical Dependency Program, Providence Hospital, Portland.

Fleming, Michael, Ph.D., clinical psychologist, Portland.

Fortner, Charles, pharmacy manager, Olympia Area, Group Health Cooperative of Puget Sound, Olympia, Washington.

Frear, Raulo, Ph.D., pharmacist, Good Samaritan Hospital, Portland.

Goodwin, Sally, executive director, Oregon Association of Homes for the Aging, Portland.

Greathouse, Joan, manager of Senior Programs, Group Health Cooperative of Puget Sound, Seattle.

Greenlick, Merwyn, MD, Ph.D., director, Kaiser Permanente Center for Health Research, Portland.

Harrington, Linda, RN, neurological nurse specialist, Microneurosurgery Consultants, Portland.

Ikehara-Martin, Greg, assistant pastor of Calvin Presbyterian Church, Tigard, Oregon.

Jampolsky, Gerald, MD, director, Center for Attitudinal Healing, Tiburon, California.

Jenkins, Lynda, RN, hospice care specialist and senior citizen health consultant, King City, Oregon.

Keaty, Charles, director of public relations, Group Health Cooperative of Puget Sound, Seattle.

Klug, Cindy, director, Project DARE (Drug and Alcohol Resources for the Elderly), Portland.

Klusky, Jay, Ph.D., stress management consultant and member of staff, Preventive Medicine Associates, Portland.

Langfitt, Virginia, RN, visiting evaluator of nursing homes for Oregon State Department of Health, King City, Oregon.

Mahan, Karen, stress management consultant and owner of BIO, a firm providing care in mentation and biofeedback, Portland.

McCann, Joseph, proprietor, McCann's Pharmacy, King City, Oregon.

McGraw, Phyllis, Ph.D., clinical psychologist, specialist in long-term care insurance for John Hancock Mutual Life Insurance Co., Portland.

Nicholson, Alison, public relations specialist, Secure Horizons (HMO), Portland.

Nonnenkamp, Lucy, Social/HMO demonstration project director, Kaiser Permanente Center for Health Research, Portland.

Olsen, George, MD, professor of pharmacology, Oregon Health Sciences University, Portland.

Olson, James, MD, general practitioner, Group Health Cooperative of Puget Sound, Seattle.

Parent, Joseph, MD, president, Preventive Medicine Associates, Portland.

Pennock, Dee, writer of syndicated medical column, King City, Oregon.

Pothetes, Leo, MA, assistant director of Project DARE (Drug and Alcohol Resources for the Elderly), Portland.

Rauscher, Elizabeth, Ph.D., assistant director, Mag-Tek Research Laboratory, Reno, Nevada.

Rosenbaum, Edward, MA, rheumatologist and author of *A Taste of My Own Medicine*, Portland.

Rosenberg, Marvin, MD, director, Senior Peer Counselor program, Group Health Cooperative of Puget Sound, Seattle.

Samuels, James, founder of The Mentat School, Portland.

Schenkel, John, MD, Dept. of Mental Health, Clackamas County, Oregon.

Schnalzer, Joan, case aide, Lehigh County Area Agency on Aging, Allentown, Pennsylvania.

Schultze, Joan, DC, Portland.

Simonson, William, Ph.D., professor of pharmacology, Oregon State College, Corvallis, Oregon.

Strother, Charles, Ph.D., former corporate president, Group Health Cooperative of Puget Sound, Seattle.

Sullivan, Dorothy, RN, director of Caring Community for Mature Adults, Lake Oswego, Oregon.

Thompson, Catherine, MD, MA, pediatrician and medical anthropologist, Portland.

Thompson, John, MD, director, Kaiser Permanente Regional Medical Laboratory, Portland.

Thornton, Betty, director, Community Services Department, Group Health Cooperative of Puget Sound, Seattle.

Ulwelling, John, executive director, Oregon State Board of Medical Examiners, Portland.

Van Bise, William, director, Mag-Tek Research Laboratory, Reno, Nevada.

Vonder Reith, John, DC, King City, Oregon.

Wart, Claire, RN, nurse-consultant to nursing homes and home care specialist with Multnomah County Public Health Dept., Portland.

Wheeler, Pam, director, Department of Senior Health Services, Good Samaritan Hospital, Portland.

Wischman, Charles, MD, general practitioner, Group Health Cooperative of Puget Sound, Seattle.